Gastrointestinal Endoscopy in Dogs and Cats

David C. Twedt, DVM
Diplomate, ACVIM

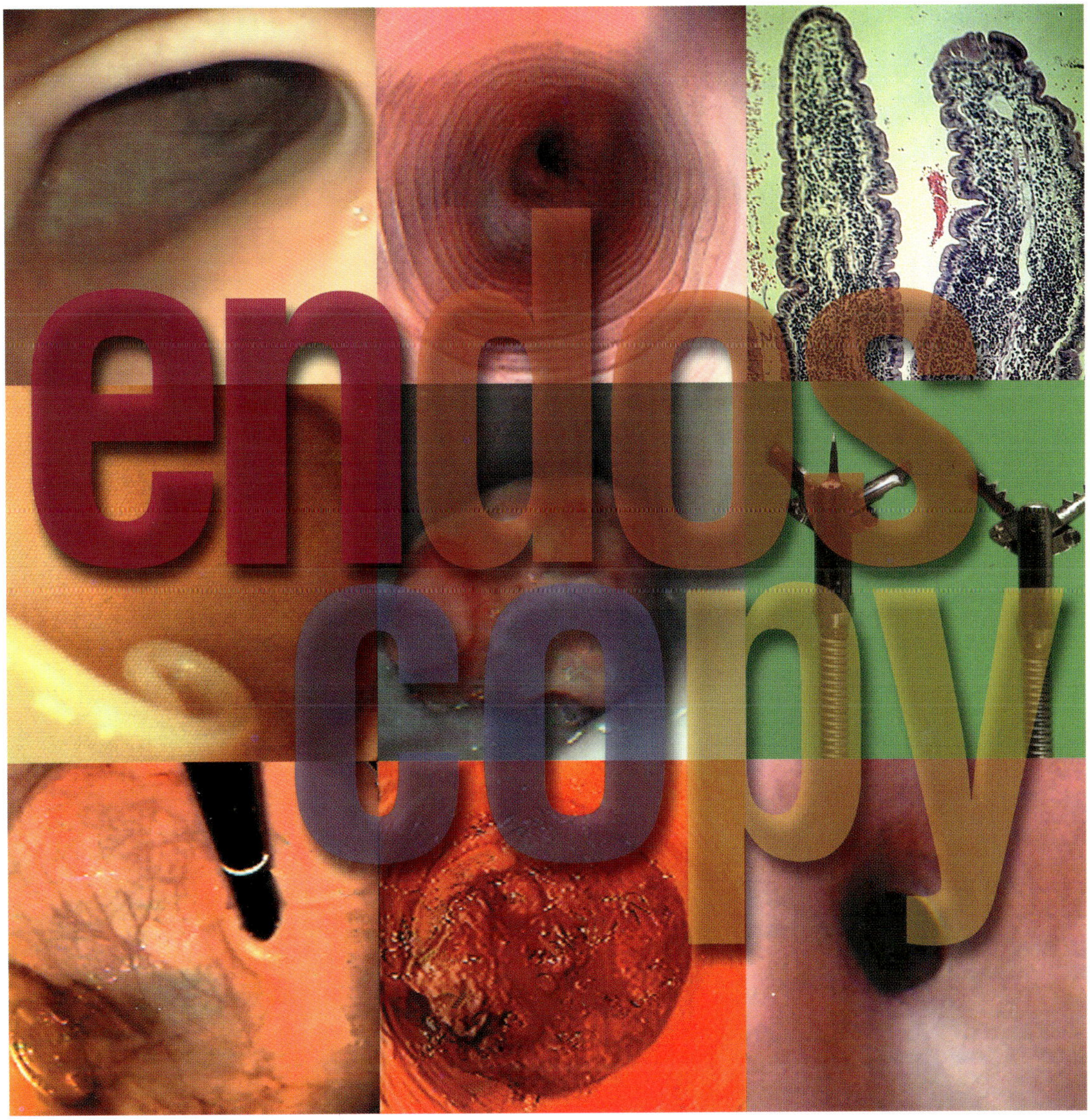

Ralston Purina Company **Clinical Handbook Series**

Published by The Gloyd Group, Inc.
Wilmington, Delaware

Printed in the United States of America.
Ralston Purina Company: Checkerboard Square, Saint Louis, Missouri, 63188
First printing, 2001.

ISBN 0-9678005-6-0

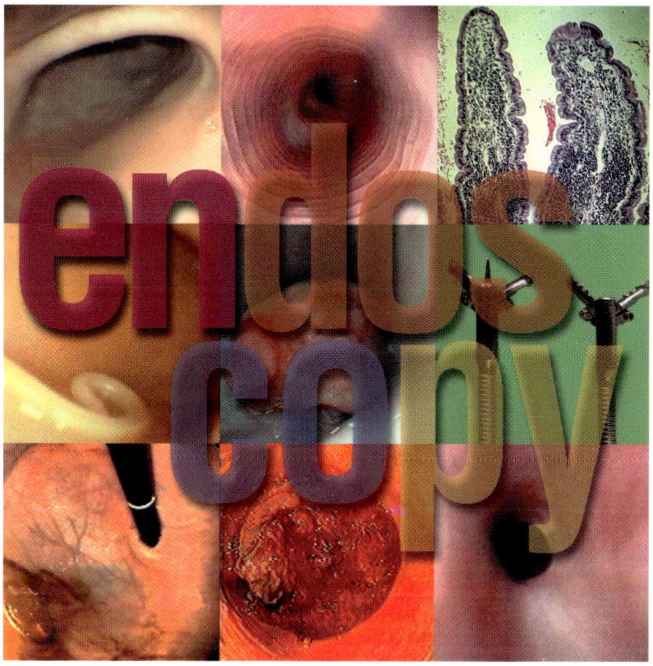

Gastrointestinal Endoscopy in Dogs and Cats

David C. Twedt, DVM
Diplomate, ACVIM

Ralston Purina Company
Clinical Handbook Series

Table of Contents

Preface

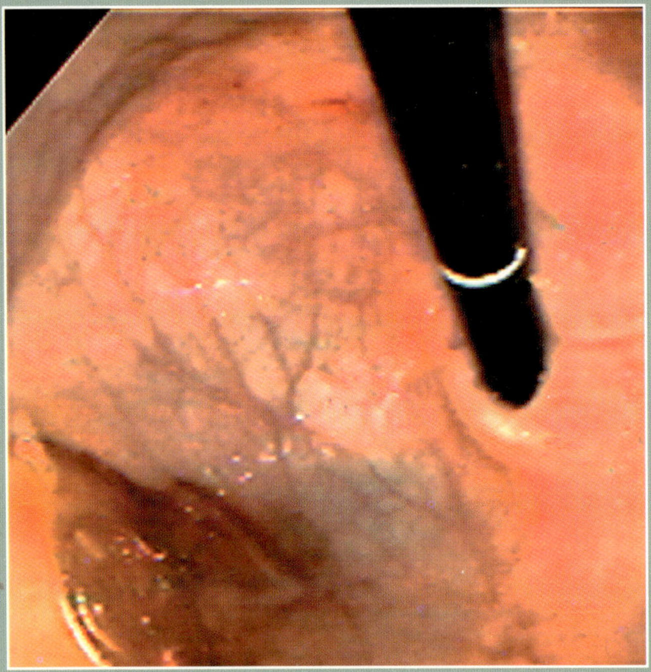

According to an old adage in medicine, "if you don't look for it, you will never diagnose it." To this end endoscopy has advanced the ability to "look for" and find abnormalities in the gastrointestinal tract. Further, endoscopy has vastly improved our understanding and capability of diagnosing gastrointestinal disease in small animals.

The author dedicates this handbook to all those that have contributed to today's knowledge of veterinary endoscopy ... with special recognition of mentor Dr. Gerald Johnson, who is the original pioneer of veterinary endoscopy. He was the first individual to perform endoscopy routinely in working up clinical cases during the early 1970s. It was Dr. Johnson's enthusiasm and teaching that kindled the author's interest in gastrointestinal endoscopy while a resident. Sincere thanks go to the many colleagues who have contributed to the author's endoscopic knowledge; to the residents who have presented constant challenges and helped him learn from his mistakes; and, perhaps, most important, to the animals that have been "scoped"—for it is from them that the author has learned the most.

The author also would like to express special thanks to his wonderful wife, Elizabeth Whitney, and son, Ryan, for their continual support over the years.

Introduction

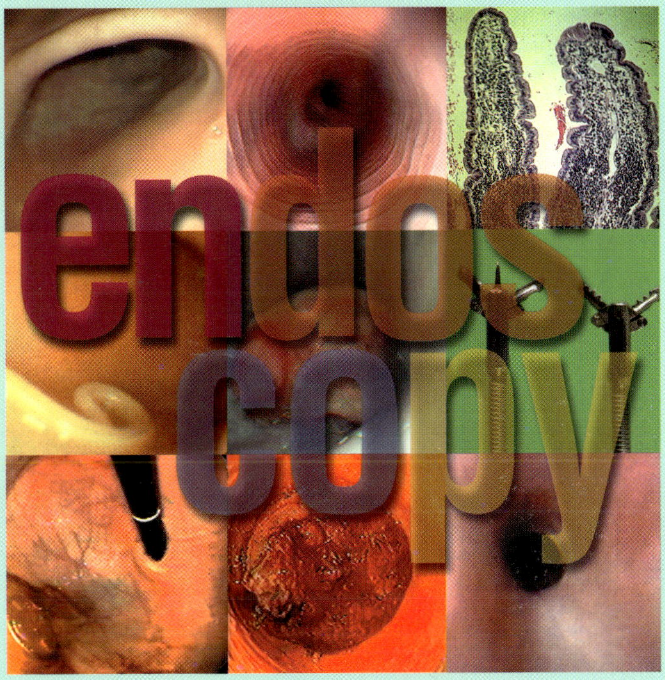

Endoscopy is an exceptionally valuable tool for the diagnosis of many small animal gastrointestinal disorders. This handbook is intended to give the reader a basic introductory overview of gastrointestinal endoscopy and to provide examples that show its diagnostic capabilities. The author recommends that those with little or no endoscopic experience learn more about the principles of endoscopy described herein by attending one of the many available continuing education endoscopy laboratories. Proficiency in endoscopic technique and interpretation comes only after many hours of practice.

Part I (Chapters 1 and 2) is designed to acquaint the reader with endoscopic basics. Included are indications, complications, and equipment requirements. It is important to understand basic endoscopic anatomy as well as the types of biopsy forceps and accessory instruments required before beginning an endoscopic procedure. These chapters include recommendations for endoscopic techniques and methods of sample collection.

Part II (Chapters 3 and 4) expands the descriptions of endoscopic findings and supports them with case studies. Chapter 3 is divided into anatomic sections corresponding to those of the gastrointestinal tract. Each of these sections describes the expected normal findings and specific techniques required for examination of that section of the gastro-intestinal tract. Also included are numerous examples of endoscopic abnormalities for each anatomic section. Chapter 4 comprises case studies that demonstrate the importance of endoscopy in the diagnosis or therapy of gastrointestinal disorders. Studying these cases can reinforce the reader's understanding of gastrointestinal disease, including when to incorporate endoscopy as a diagnostic tool.

Part III contains an **Index of Figures** that describes all of the endoscopic images and other photographs presented in this handbook. In addition, a **Glossary of Terms** highlights useful definitions, as they relate to gastrointestinal endoscopy. The **Suggested Reading** section lists additional resources that cover topics in small animal gastrointestinal endoscopy, including references on basic endoscopy as well articles that describe the disease syndromes presented in Part II.

Part I

Chapter 1: **Endoscopic Basics— Indications and Equipment**

Gastrointestinal endoscopy for small animals has evolved to become both an important diagnostic option and, in some situations, even a therapeutic solution. Once considered to be only an adjunct to other diagnostic means, gastrointestinal endoscopy is now one of the most important techniques for evaluating patients with gastrointestinal signs. The minimal invasiveness, the increasing diagnostic capabilities, and the professional enjoyment in performing endoscopic procedures all add to the popularity of endoscopy in small animal practice. Historically, gastrointestinal endoscopes were only found in teaching hospitals or large referral centers. Today they are available in many small animal private practices throughout the world.

Endoscopy lends itself to a role in gastrointestinal evaluation because it provides visual documentation of the gastrointestinal lumen and the ability to collect samples for analysis, remove foreign bodies, or perform such therapeutic procedures as esophageal stricture dilation. Often other diagnostic tests, such as barium contrast studies or ultrasound evaluation of the gastrointestinal tract, may not be sensitive enough to delineate many gastrointestinal mucosal disorders and fail to provide a means of collecting tissue for analysis. Also current laboratory tests for gastrointestinal disease are variable in their diagnostic sensitivity.

Further, endoscopy offers the advantage of enabling visual examination of a mucosal surface and the ability to obtain mucosal biopsies for histologic examination or fluid aspiration for analysis or culture. The potential limitation of gastrointestinal endoscopy is the inability to diagnose submucosal lesions, gastrointestinal motility disorders, or lesions that cannot be reached by the endoscope.

General indications for gastrointestinal endoscopy include investigation of unexplained gastrointestinal-related signs (***Table 1***). Endoscopy is usually performed when a patient shows clinical signs or there is laboratory, radiographic, or ultrasound evidence of esophageal, gastric, duodenal, or colonic abnormalities. Esophageal and gastric foreign body removal with an endoscope is now preferred to surgical intervention because of the minimal invasiveness of the procedure. Endoscopes are also used for gastrostomy tube placement.

Occasionally, occult disease is diagnosed using endoscopy. For example, the author has observed animals that presented with only the complaint of anorexia yet, even after a comprehensive evaluation, no diagnosis could be made. Following endoscopy in these cases, it was possible to identify gastric adenocarcinoma as the cause for the unexplained anorexia. Specific indications for evaluation of each segment of the gastrointestinal tract are described in Part II of this handbook.

It is important to realize that there are limitations associated with gastrointestinal endoscopy. These are based, in part, on the physical characteristics of the scope—both diameter and insertion tube length—and on the size of the animal being examined. The length of the endoscope is a limiting factor in how far the scope can be passed through the small intestine. Size and depth of biopsies taken from the gastrointestinal wall are also limited. Sample taking is generally confined to the mucosa, consequently submucosal or deeper lesions are missed. There is also some restriction in the size of gastrointestinal foreign bodies that can be removed relative to the shape of the foreign object and the type of grasping forceps available.

Complications associated with gastrointestinal endoscopy are rare. Although endoscopy is considered to be a minimally invasive procedure, it does require general anesthesia in the patient. Organ perforation is a dreaded potential complication but is extremely rare as long as the basic principles of endoscopy are followed. The most common endoscopic complication is a consequence of overdistention

TABLE 1. SOME COMMON INDICATIONS FOR GASTROINTESTINAL ENDOSCOPY

Clinical Signs		
Anorexia	Hematemesis	Retching
Constipation	Hematochezia	Salivation
Diarrhea	Melena	Tenesmus
Dyschezia	Mucoid feces	Vomiting
Dysphagia	Nausea	Weight loss
	Regurgitation	

of the stomach with insufflated air. Excessive gaseous distention of the stomach can result in hypotension and compromise respiratory function. This problem is prevented by constant awareness of the degree of gastric distention being caused by air.

Endoscopic Equipment

Gastrointestinal Endoscopes

The basic gastrointestinal endoscope system consists of two components: the **fiberoptic endoscope** and a **light source.** Fiberoptics in the endoscope are simply bundles of tiny glass fibers that function in transporting either light for illumination or for transmitting images. To enable image transmission, the very small-diameter glass fibers are coherently packed into bundles that transmit an image to the eyepiece in the endoscope. Although each fiber produces only an extremely tiny point of uniform light and color, when the fibers are viewed together as a unit, an image is observed.

The size of individual fibers, compactness of fiber bundles, and accuracy of coherent bundle relationship determine the sharpness of the image. Fiber bundles are quite fragile, however, and can be damaged by improper handling. If a glass fiber is broken, then it will not transmit light and is seen as a black dot when looking through the viewing lens. The lens system at the proximal end of the image bundle magnifies the image for operator viewing. A video camera can also be attached to the eyepiece and the image viewed on a video monitor.

Illumination fiberoptics are randomly grouped glass fibers that transmit light originating from a high-intensity light source housed outside the patient. The light source that illuminates the endoscope is either a halogen or the preferred xenon light.

Newer gastrointestinal video endoscopes incorporate the same illumination fiberoptics used previously, but the image is recorded by a small microelectric video chip located in the distal tip of the endoscope. The image is then transmitted electronically to a video processor and viewed on a television monitor. These later model endoscopes provide superior images but are also more costly.

Endoscope Anatomy

A basic fiberoptic endoscope consists of three sections: the **insertion tube,** the **handpiece,** and the **umbilical cord** (*Figure 1.1*).

The **insertion tube** is the portion of the endoscope that passes into the gastrointestinal tract. It is generally 100 cm

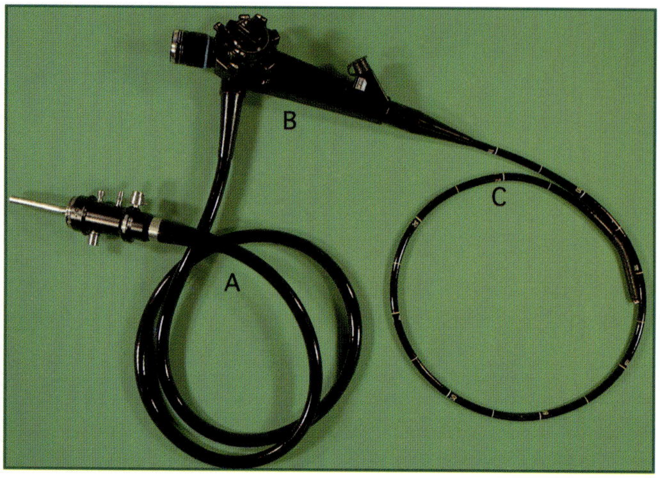

Figure 1.1 Typical gastrointestinal endoscope showing (A) the umbilical cord, which is attached to a light source; (B) the handpiece containing the control knobs and valves; and (C) the insertion tube.

or longer, flexible, and contains the image and illumination fiberoptics. Within the insertion tube is an insufflation and water channel through which air can be blown into the gastrointestinal tract to distend the lumen or water can pass to clean the distal viewing lens. A second suction-biopsy channel permits aspiration of air or fluid and enables passage of a biopsy forceps or other instruments. The distal tip of the gastrointestinal endoscope moves in four planes of deflection. Most endoscopes have the ability to deflect in one plane, at least 180° or greater deflection.

The **handpiece** is the portion of the endoscope that contains the control mechanism and houses the eyepiece for visualization. Deflection knobs in the handpiece are used for up/down angulation and right/left angulation of the distal tip. On most endoscopes, these knobs have locks to maintain their position. Although rarely necessary to use during small animal endoscopy, the lock system can provide an endoscopist with the ability to maintain a desired position of the distal tip for biopsy or other manipulations. An air/water valve is also located in the handpiece. When the valve is occluded, air is passed through the insertion tube for insufflation of the lumen. Depression of the air/water valve results in water passage for the purpose of cleaning the viewing lens. Depression of the suction valve results in suction of air or fluid through the operation channel. There is a separate operating channel opening in which a forceps or other instruments can be passed. It should be noted that suction is not possible when instruments are in the operating channel.

The **umbilical cord** of the endoscope conveys light from the external light source through illumination fiberoptics.

Endoscopy requires either a high-intensity halogen or a xenon external light source. Higher wattages provide greater illumination. Endoscopic light sources also contain an air pump, which is necessary for insufflation. A separate vacuum source is necessary for suction through the endoscope and is not part of the endoscopic light source system.

Video endoscopy can be performed by attaching a specialized video camera to the endoscope eyepiece or by using a video endoscope that has a built-in microchip camera at the distal insertion tube. With either setup, the image is viewed on a video monitor. Image documentation can be obtained by using a video recorder or video printer.

Endoscope Selection

Selecting the perfect small animal gastrointestinal endoscope can be a difficult proposition. Many makes and sizes of endoscopes are available, but there is no one endoscope that appears to be ideal for all endoscopic procedures (ie, gastrointestinal endoscopy, bronchoscopy, nasal endoscopy, cystoscopy, laparoscopy, and reproductive endoscopy). The key factors in selecting a gastrointestinal endoscope are: insertion tube length, diameter, biopsy channel size, and scope quality and cost. Another factor that should be considered is the type of examinations to be performed. For example, an exclusively feline practice has different endoscopic length and diameter requirements from those in a small animal practice that deals with predominately large-breed dogs.

Currently available human gastrointestinal endoscopes generally have insertion-tube lengths of approximately 110 cm and diameters ranging from 7.9 to 12 mm. The smaller diameters and length are suitable for cats and small dogs and make entry through the pylorus easier. However, when dealing with larger dogs, the human endoscopes that are 110 cm in length may be too short to enter the duodenum. Endoscopes with an outer diameter of greater than 10 mm should also be avoided to prevent difficulty entering the pylorus.

Several veterinary endoscopes now produced feature smaller diameters (7 to 9 mm), and most have longer insertion tube lengths ranging from 125 to 150 cm. These endoscopes are better suited to use in the large dog but can be easily used in the small patient as well. The long insertion tube length of these newer endoscopes sometimes makes the endoscopic procedure cumbersome in a very small patient. A disadvantage of the smaller-diameter (7 to 8 mm) endoscopes is their smaller-diameter biopsy channel (approximately 2.2 mm). Larger-diameter scopes generally have a 2.8-mm biopsy channel accommodating a larger biopsy forceps, hence, permitting retrieval of greater biopsy samples.

Endoscopic Instruments

A number of flexible instruments are available for use with an endoscope. Basic instruments suggested for small animal endoscopy include a biopsy forceps, foreign-body grasping instruments, cytology brushes, and aspiration tubes (***Figure 1.2***). Other available instruments include snares, baskets, injection needles, and coagulation electrodes. All of these instruments are available as either reusable or single-use disposables. When using any type of endoscopic instrument, it is important to ensure compatibility with the associated endoscope.

There are several types of biopsy forceps available for endoscopes. The most common forceps used is either the oval cup forceps or the oval cup with alligator teeth (***Figure 1.3***). Controversy exists as to which type produces

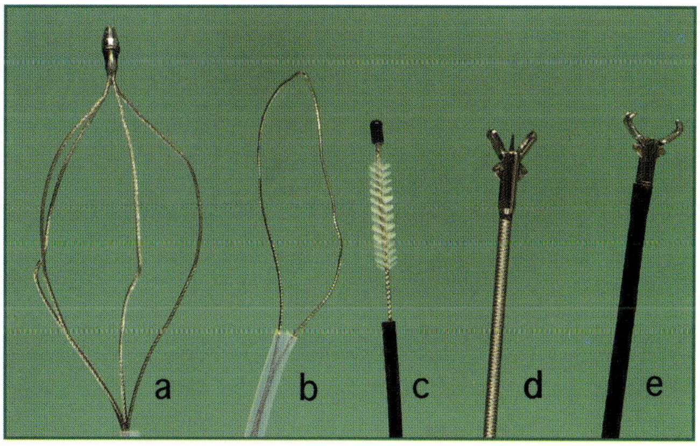

Figure 1.2 Examples of basic endoscopic instruments: (a) wire basket, (b) wire snare, (c) cytology brush, (d) foreign body grasper with spike, and (e) foreign body grasper.

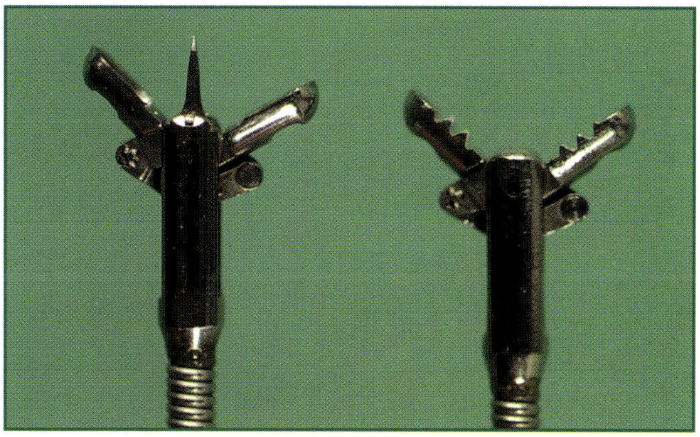

Figure 1.3 Two types of biopsy forceps: oval cups with a spike (left) and alligator cups (right).

the best biopsy sample; however, some endoscopists believe the alligator type is superior at yielding a larger biopsy sample size. Either type of forceps can be obtained with a central spike within the cups, which is helpful in preventing the forceps from sliding down the mucosa during biopsy. Biopsy forceps should always be kept clean, sharp, and well lubricated. A biopsy forceps should never be used for foreign body retrieval, because, once dull, it is difficult to obtain adequate tissue samples.

It is also recommended to have several foreign body retrieval instruments. Suggestions include a two- or three-pronged grasping forceps and a foreign body retrieval wire basket or snare. With these two instruments, most foreign bodies can be removed. Brushes used to obtain cytologic samples are helpful in many cases, as are aspiration tubes for fluid collection.

Chapter 2: **Technique and Sample Collection**

Equipment Setup and Patient Preparation

A designated space should be identified for gastrointestinal endoscopy. The endoscopic area should be large enough to accommodate an anesthesia machine, endoscopy equipment, and the operator and assistant (***Figure 2.1***). Adjustable room lighting is helpful because endoscopic images are best viewed in a darkened environment. An endoscopic cart is recommended to hold the light source, monitors, video printers, and other equipment. Use of a cart makes the endoscope unit portable and, thus, more versatile. The patient is usually placed on an adjustable table or wet table. Construction of a storage cabinet within the endoscopy room is a convenient and safe way to store the endoscope and instruments (***Figure 2.2***). It is strongly recommended that endoscopes be stored in a hanging position to permit adequate drying. Storing an endoscope in the suitcase that is used for transport is not recommended.

Before performing upper gastrointestinal endoscopy, the patient is fasted for at least 12 to 24 hours. This restriction is important because the presence of food in the stomach makes gastric evaluation almost impossible. It should be noted that patients with gastric disease often have altered motility, and a standard 12-hour fast may be insufficient. For colonoscopy, adequate bowel preparation is essential and is discussed in Chapter 3 under "Colonoscopy, Technique."

General anesthesia with a cuffed endotracheal tube is recommended for all endoscopic procedures. This setup prevents damage to the endoscope and prevents the chance of aspiration. An oral speculum must always be used to prevent the patient from biting the endoscope.

For routine upper or lower endoscopy, the patient is placed in left lateral recumbency. In this position, the pylorus is best visualized and the duodenum most easily entered. The operator should stand directly in front of the patient facing the mouth. When using video endoscopy, the monitor should be placed in such a position that the operator looks directly at the screen. This positioning maintains orientation of the endoscope image, the operator, and video monitor. Maintaining this special relationship is important because, when the endoscope control knobs are deflected (up/down or left/right), the same direction of movement is viewed on the monitor.

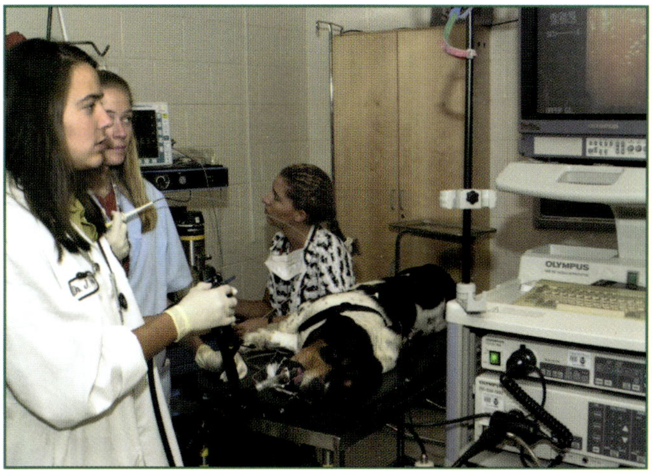

Figure 2.1 The veterinary endoscopy room at Colorado State University showing the endoscopic equipment, patient, and technicians assisting the endoscopist.

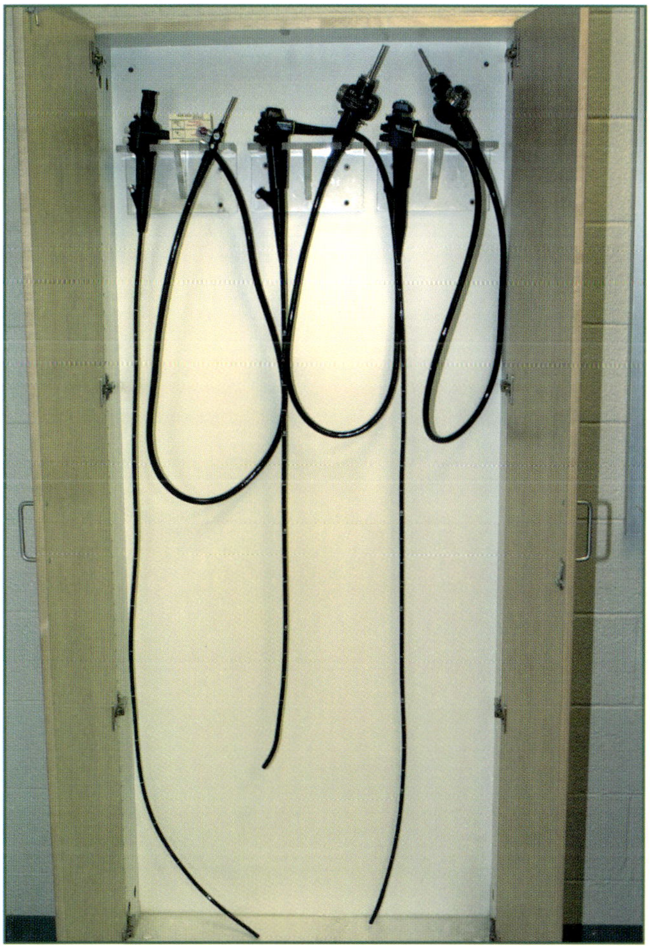

Figure 2.2 Endoscopic storage cabinet recommended for optimum storage of endoscopes and instruments.

Correct Use of the Endoscope

The endoscope handpiece is held in the left hand with the light cable cradled in the crux between the thumb and forefinger. The left index finger is used to depress the air/water and suction valves (***Figure 2.3***). Many endoscopists use the left thumb to maneuver the up/down control knob; however, this movement is more difficult for operators that have small hands. The right hand is used to deflect the left/right control knob, to advance the insertion tube, and to advance endoscopic instruments. It is helpful to have the endoscopic assistant hold and aid in advancing the insertion tube, leaving the endoscopist's right hand free to adjust the control knobs. To maintain orientation, it is important to attempt to keep the endoscope as straight as possible. In some situations slight torque can be applied to the insertion tube if the four-way directional control does not move the endoscope tip to the desired area to be viewed. Care should be taken not to apply undue torque or pressure, which could damage the endoscope.

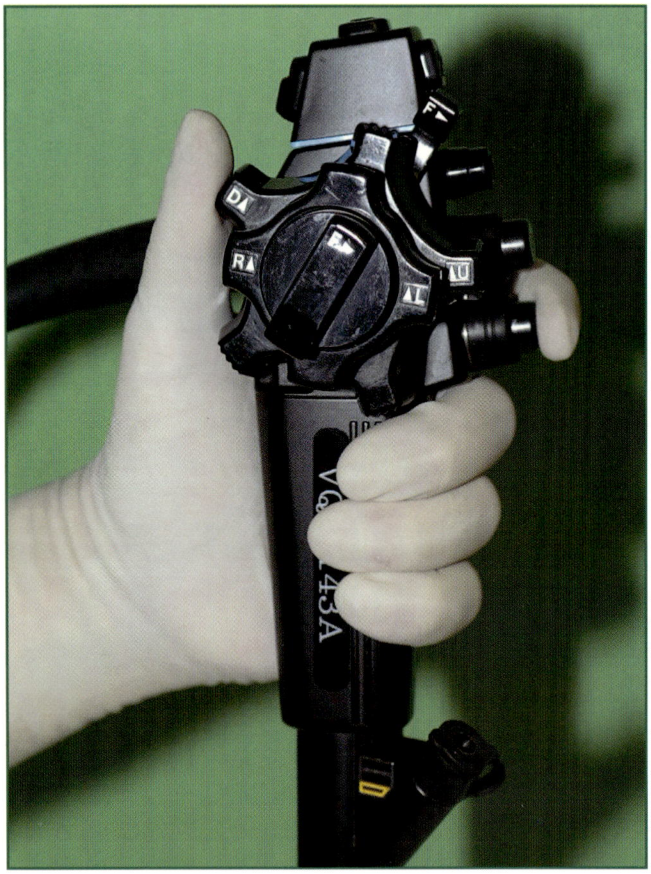

Figure 2.3 Recommended method of holding the endoscope handpiece. The umbilical cord is held between the thumb and forefinger. The thumb maneuvers the up/down control knob. The forefinger controls the air/water and suction valves. (The right hand controls the left/right control knob.)

Several general rules of endoscopy are applicable to every endoscopic procedure. First, the endoscopist should not advance the endoscope blindly without viewing the lumen. Second, the endoscope or endoscopic forceps should never be forced with undue pressure. Finally, if the endoscopist becomes "lost" during endoscopy, then the endoscope should be withdrawn until orientation is regained. At the conclusion of endoscopy, the lumen is deflated and the endoscope is removed. If refluxed gastric fluid is present in the esophagus, it should be removed to prevent secondary esophagitis.

"RULES" OF ENDOSCOPY

- Always be sure the lumen is visible during advancement of the endoscope.
- Never use undue pressure to force the endoscope or an endoscopic forceps.
- If orientation is "lost" during an endoscopic procedure, withdraw the endoscope until correct orientation is regained.

Sample Collection

Mucosal biopsies are generally acquired whenever a dog or cat is undergoing endoscopy. When taking biopsy specimens, the forceps should be directed as perpendicularly as possible to the tissue, the tissue pinched, and the forceps then pulled away. If the forceps is not directly perpendicular, it may slide along the tissue and often yields inadequate samples. Using a biopsy forceps with a spike helps prevent the forceps from sliding. To aid in performing the biopsy technique, it is advisable to deflate the lumen slightly to reduce the mucosal tension, thereby allowing greater grasp of the mucosa. Generally, five to seven samples should be obtained from each anatomic area under investigation.

The tissue obtained through biopsy can also be used for impression smear cytology, culture, or for histopathology. Because of the small sample size, prior discussion with the pathologist regarding the best method of sample submission is advisable. Some laboratories provide small plastic cassettes in which to place the samples (***Figure 2.4***). An alternative method is to place the samples on a saline-moistened piece of lens cleaning paper. When all of the samples have been collected, the paper holding the samples is gently wrapped and placed in formalin.

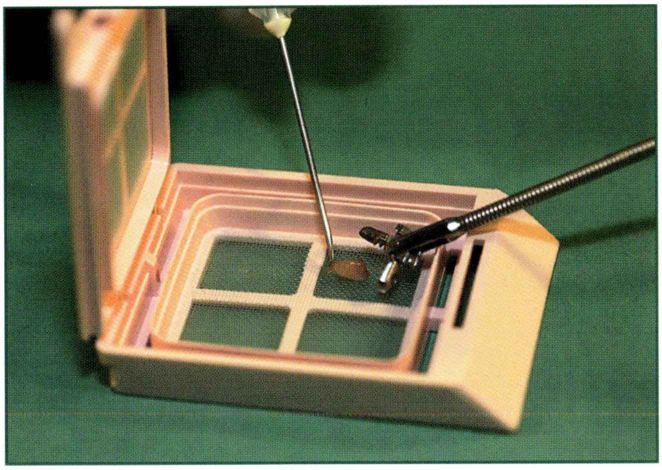

Figure 2.4 Biopsy sample being placed in a histopathology cassette. A needle is used to carefully remove the tissue from the forceps. When all samples have been collected, the cassette is closed and placed in formalin.

Brush cytology samples are obtained by using a special cytology brush. The area to be examined is gently brushed, and the bristles are then rolled on a clean microscope slide, which is submitted for cytologic evaluation. This technique has proven to be a useful adjunct to endoscopic biopsy and histology. Cytology may provide additional diagnostic information, especially relating to such superficial material as bacteria, protozoa, and parasites, which may be lost in the processing of tissue samples for histology. Endoscopically collected cytology results often correlate with histologic findings of inflammatory or neoplastic lesions. Using an aspiration tube, luminal fluid can also be collected for cytologic examination or culture.

Part II

Chapter 3: **Endoscopic Findings—Esophagus, Stomach, Intestine, and Colon**

The Esophagus

Endoscopy of the esophagus begins with the patient's head and neck extended. The endoscope is passed through the oral pharynx and into the upper esophageal sphincter. Resistance may be encountered if the scope is directed into one of the piriform recesses that are located on either side of the larynx. After the scope is in the proximal body of the esophagus, the lumen is then insufflated with air.

The endoscope should not be advanced without visualization of the lumen. If the lumen does not distend following insufflation, manual compression of the esophagus just below the larynx prevents air from escaping around the upper esophageal sphincter. Animals with a potential esophageal perforation, such as could occur from foreign bodies, should be endoscoped with caution. Insufflation of a perforated esophagus results in air movement into the chest cavity causing a tension pneumothorax.

A normal esophagus is whitish-pink and glistening with mucus over the surface (***Figure 3.1***). Impressions of the trachea lying adjacent to the esophagus in the cervical area can be seen as the lumen is distended with air. As the endoscope is advanced into the thoracic esophagus, pulsation of the aorta and heart against the esophageal wall becomes visible. The esophagus should distend easily and the longitudinal folds flatten and become smooth. There should be little fluid within the lumen, other than a small amount of swallowed saliva.

The distal esophagus of the cat contains smooth muscle and is seen endoscopically as a series of circular striations (sometimes referred to as a herringbone esophagus) extending to the lower esophageal sphincter (***Figure 3.2***). Submucosal blood vessels are also visible in the distal esophagus of cats but are not as apparent in dogs.

In a normal animal, the lower esophageal sphincter (LES) is generally closed (***Figure 3.3***). At the LES, there is a demarcation between the esophageal and gastric mucosa, where the redder color of the gastric mucosa is often evident extending into the LES. This juncture is referred to as the gastric rosette. A dilated or open LES, although sometimes normal, could suggest a gastroesophageal reflux disorder, especially if concurrent distal esophagitis is present.

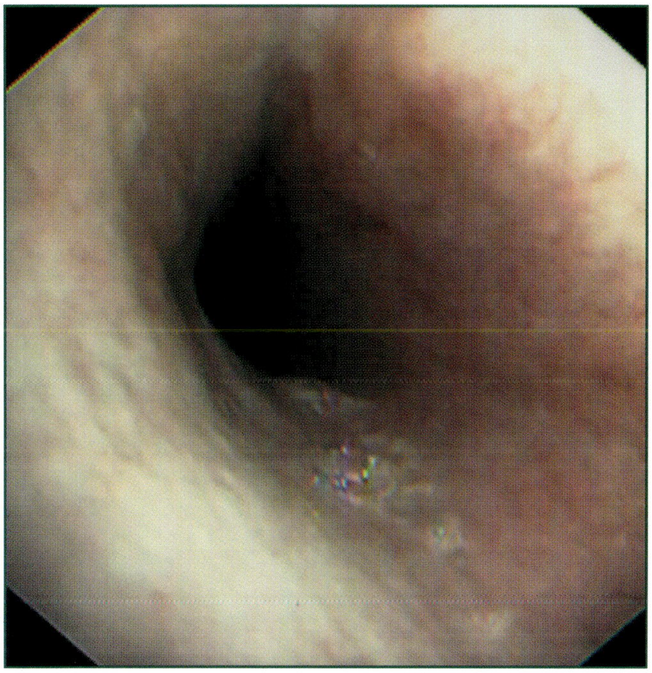

Figure 3.1 Normal cervical esophagus in a dog.

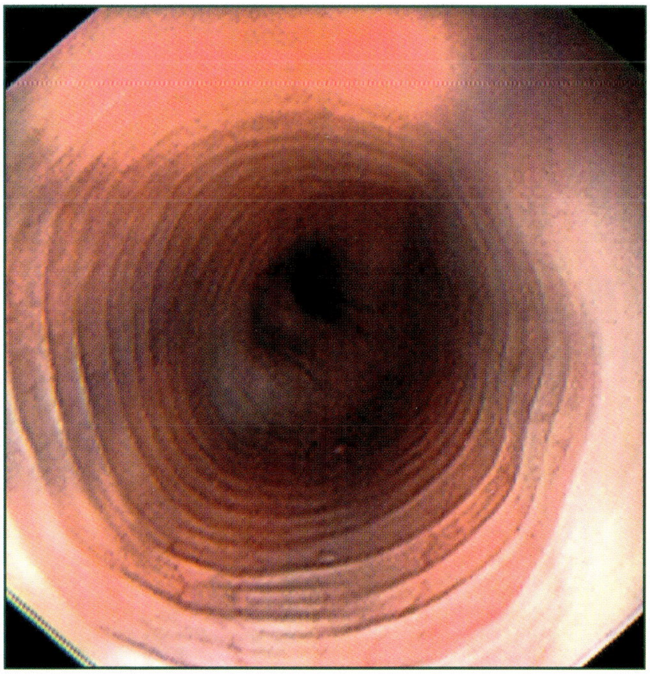

Figure 3.2 Normal feline distal esophagus showing circular striations of the smooth muscle and prominent submucosal blood vessels.

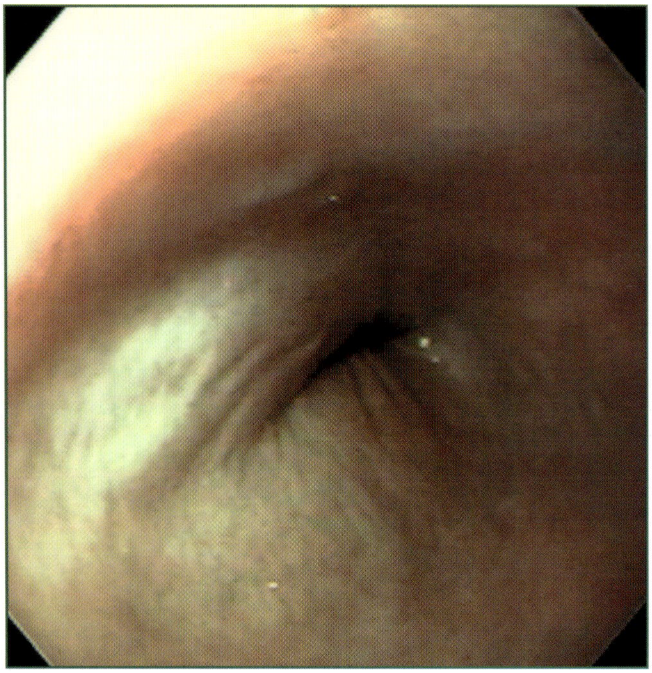

Figure 3.3 Normal canine lower esophageal sphincter.

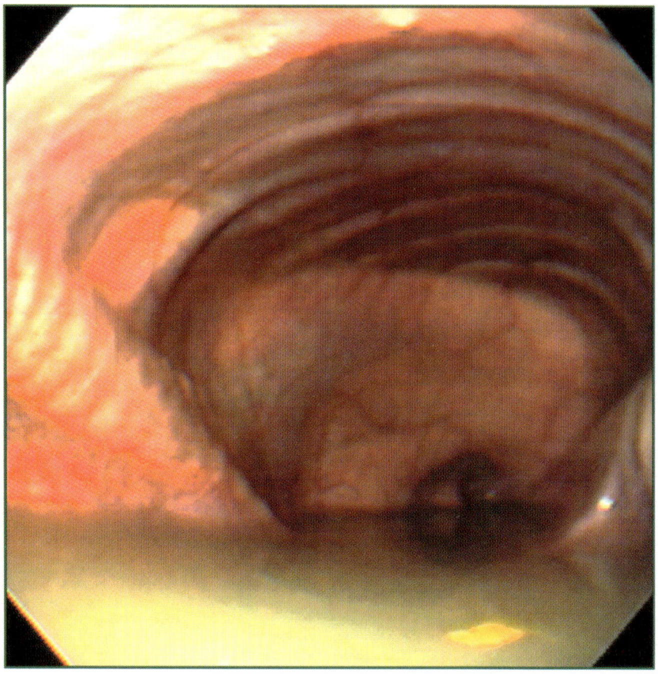

Figure 3.4 Idiopathic canine megaesophagus showing marked esophageal dilation and fluid within the lumen. Imprints of the trachea and ribs can be seen.

Biopsy of the esophageal mucosa is difficult because of the tough characteristics of the stratified squamous epithelium. As a result of the difficulty in esophageal biopsy, the diagnosis of inflammatory changes in the esophagus is frequently made through visual inspection alone.

Esophageal Abnormalities

Megaesophagus

Although megaesophagus is one of the most common esophageal disorders in dogs, endoscopy may not be helpful in making the diagnosis because the esophagus is normally dilated during insufflation. In cases of idiopathic megaesophagus, however, marked dilation of the lumen greater than occurs during routine endoscopy is often seen (***Figure 3.4***).

Generally, the diagnosis of esophageal motility disorders is best made using contrast radiology. Endoscopy does help determine if secondary esophagitis is present and is useful in ruling out obstructive disease that could also cause esophageal dilatation. Care should be taken when endoscopically evaluating a patient with a megaesophagus because of the potential for secondary aspiration pneumonia. Endoscopy is sometimes performed to place a gastrostomy tube as a means of providing nutrition for certain patients with megaesophagus.

Esophageal Foreign Bodies

When the diagnosis is an esophageal foreign body, prompt removal is required because the longer the foreign body remains in the esophagus, the more mucosal damage occurs. Bones are the most common esophageal foreign bodies found in dogs. Bone foreign bodies usually lodge in the distal esophagus, with lodging at the heart base the next most frequent site and lodging at the thoracic inlet rare. Removal of esophageal foreign bodies involves using either rigid or flexible fiberoptic endoscopes. Most esophageal foreign bodies can be removed with various grasping forceps, wire baskets, or snares.

The disadvantage of using a gastrointestinal fiberoptic endoscope is the small size of foreign-body grasping instruments that can be used. Removal of large foreign bodies, such as bones, often requires a large, rigid esophageal scope and a pronged grasping forceps. The advantage of a rigid endoscopic tube is that it mechanically dilates the esophagus, and the endoscopist can pass a larger-sized grasping forceps through the rigid esophageal scope to retrieve the foreign body. In cases where large bones or other foreign bodies cannot be retrieved orally, the endoscopist may find it necessary to attempt to push them into the stomach. It is much safer to surgically remove foreign bodies from the stomach than from the esophagus.

Generally, bones pushed into the stomach can be left there, as they will undergo digestion. Following endoscopic removal of a foreign body, the esophagus should be carefully evaluated. Lacerations that do not extend through the esophageal wall and small perforations usually heal without complications. Full-thickness tears or large areas of necrosis often require surgical intervention.

Esophagitis

Esophagitis can result from direct mechanical trauma, ingestion of toxic substances, or reflux of gastric acid. The physical appearance associated with esophagitis includes erythema, erosions, and mucosal irregularity. There may be copious amounts of saliva and mucus, sometimes containing blood within the lumen. The diagnosis of gastroesophageal reflux (reflux esophagitis) is best made using endoscopy.

In most, but not all, normal dogs or cats, the LES should be closed; however, identifying a large, open LES during endoscopy—in conjunction with a reddened hyperemic distal esophageal mucosa—is consistent with gastroesophageal reflux. Friable or ulcerated mucosa in the distal esophagus with pooling of gastric fluid within the lumen should alert the endoscopist to the possibility of this disorder.

Esophageal Strictures

Esophageal strictures are commonly associated with direct mucosal trauma or reflux of gastric acid. Strictures may occur as narrow fibrous bands or as long segmental lesions. Contrast studies using barium or barium-food mixtures can demonstrate esophageal narrowing. Intramural strictures should not be confused with vascular ring anomalies, periesophageal masses, or intraluminal masses. Endoscopy provides the best means of identifying the presence and character of most intraluminal strictures.

A stricture in the esophagus is best treated using balloon catheters that are advanced into the constriction under endoscopic control. After it is within the stricture, the balloon is inflated under pressure to dilate the stricture radially. The dilation procedure is repeated, using increasingly larger balloon catheters, until adequate esophageal dilation is achieved.

Vascular Ring Anomalies

A vascular ring anomaly results from malformation of one of the great vessels that entraps the esophagus and causes clinical signs of esophageal obstruction. In some situations it is difficult to differentiate an inflammatory stricture from a vascular ring anomaly. The diagnosis of a vascular ring anomaly is routinely made using barium contrast radiographs demonstrating esophageal dilation cranial to the base of the heart. Endoscopy becomes helpful in confirming the diagnosis of extraluminal compression of the esophagus by large blood vessels (***Figure 3.5***).

Esophageal Neoplasia

Neoplasia is uncommon in the esophagus and accounts for less than 0.5 percent of all cancer diagnosed in dogs and cats. Esophageal neoplasia may arise either as primary esophageal in origin or as a periesophageal mass or metastatic esophageal lesions (***Figure 3.6***). Leiomyomas are the most common benign tumors of the esophagus. They are usually observed as incidental findings unless they are large enough to obstruct the esophageal lumen. Leiomyomas most often arise in the area of the LES. Esophageal papillomas are benign tumors that occasionally occur in the esophagus and are possibly the result of chronic inflammatory changes.

Squamous cell carcinoma is the most common primary malignant esophageal neoplasm in cats. It occurs more commonly in older females and is located in the middle third of the esophagus, just caudal to the thoracic inlet.

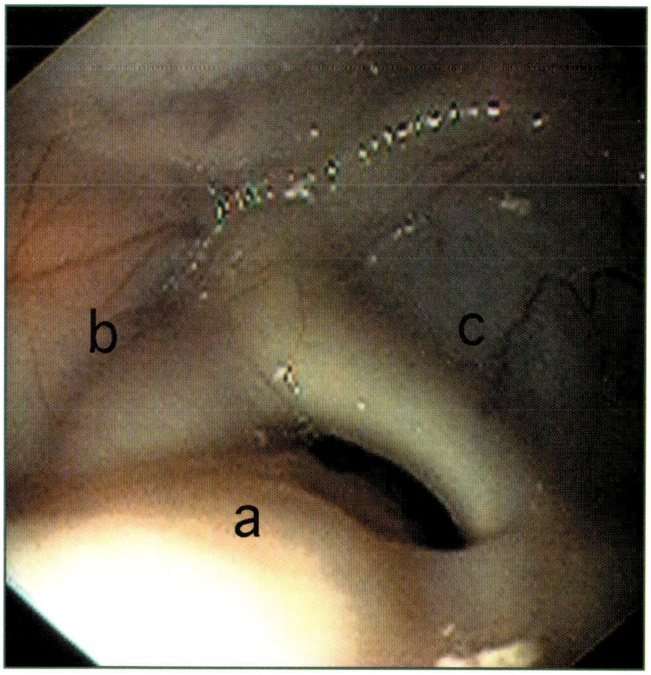

Figure 3.5 Vascular ring anomaly in a dog from a persistent right aortic arch showing narrowing of the esophageal lumen: (a) trachea, (b) aorta, and (c) persistent right aortic arch.

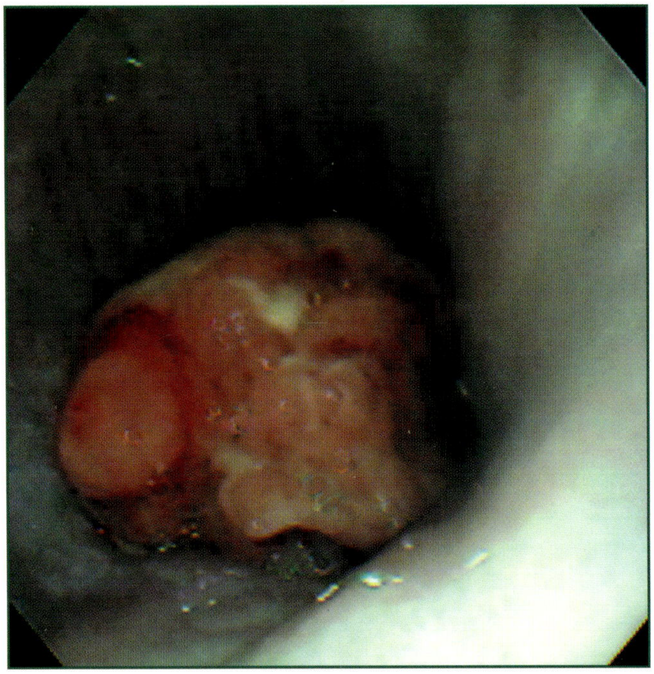

Figure 3.6 Adenocarcinoma arising in the distal esophagus of a dog.

Esophagoscopy enables visual evaluation of the esophageal lumen and the opportunity to obtain a mucosal biopsy.

Hiatal Hernia

The most common type of hiatal hernia found in dogs and cats is a sliding hiatal hernia, which is defined as cranial displacement of the abdominal esophagus, gastroesophageal junction (GEJ), and a portion of the stomach through a large, loose esophageal hiatus. Herniation is usually intermittent and signs are related to reflux esophagitis. Diagnosis of disorders of the GEJ is generally made using radiology. Survey radiographs may demonstrate esophageal dilation and an increased density in the distal esophagus from the GEJ and stomach within the caudal esophagus.

Barium contrast studies are generally required to diagnose a sliding hiatal hernia. The diagnosis is confirmed by demonstrating cranial displacement of the gastroesophageal junction and stomach into the caudal thoracic mediastinum. As hiatal herniation is often intermittent, radiology may fail to demonstrate a hiatal hernia. Endoscopy, however, provides additional evidence of a sliding hiatal hernia. Evidence of reflux esophagitis with an open LES supports the diagnosis.

Further documentation is obtained when the endoscope is passed into the stomach and retroflexed to view the LES from the gastric side. When the stomach is insufflated with air, there may be cranial displacement of the lower esophageal sphincter and cardiac region of the stomach through a weakened or enlarged esophageal hiatus in the diaphragm. Impressions made by the borders of an enlarged esophageal hiatus can be seen on the gastric cardia. Observing cranial LES displacement and a large esophageal hiatus with appropriate clinical signs is suggestive of a sliding hiatal hernia.

Esophageal Diverticula

Diverticula occur as saclike dilatations or outpouching of mucosa through one or more layers of the esophageal wall. They are generally secondary results of damage to the mucosal wall by foreign bodies. The consequences of diverticula are disturbances of normal esophageal motility and accumulation of food and fluid within the diverticulum. Small lesions may be asymptomatic, while large ones usually result in significant clinical signs associated with distress after eating. Signs include odynophagia, salivation, retching, and regurgitation. Ataxia, walking stiffly, and vague signs of discomfort have also been described in dogs with diverticula. Some diverticula may progress to severe esophageal impaction and ultimate perforation, with resultant signs of mediastinitis and respiratory disease.

Gastric Evaluation

Endoscopic Technique

Endoscopic examination of the stomach should begin with the patient in left lateral recumbency. The antrum and pylorus are best evaluated with the animal in that position because it places them in a superior abdominal location away from the pressure of adjacent organs. It is also the position from which the duodenum is most easily entered.

Following examination of the esophagus, the tip of the endoscope is directed through the lumen of the lower esophageal sphincter and then gently passed into the stomach. The endoscopist can easily distinguish between gastric mucosa and esophageal mucosa, as the stomach is redder and gastric rugae are generally evident. Following entry into the stomach, the tip of the endoscope is usually facing the greater curvature of the stomach (***Figure 3.7***). At this point, the lumen of the stomach should carefully be insufflated with air. As the lumen distends, the gastric rugae begin to flatten. The amount of insufflation should be only enough to enable viewing the lumen.

Overdistention should be avoided for several reasons. Gastric overdistention can result in cardiopulmonary com-

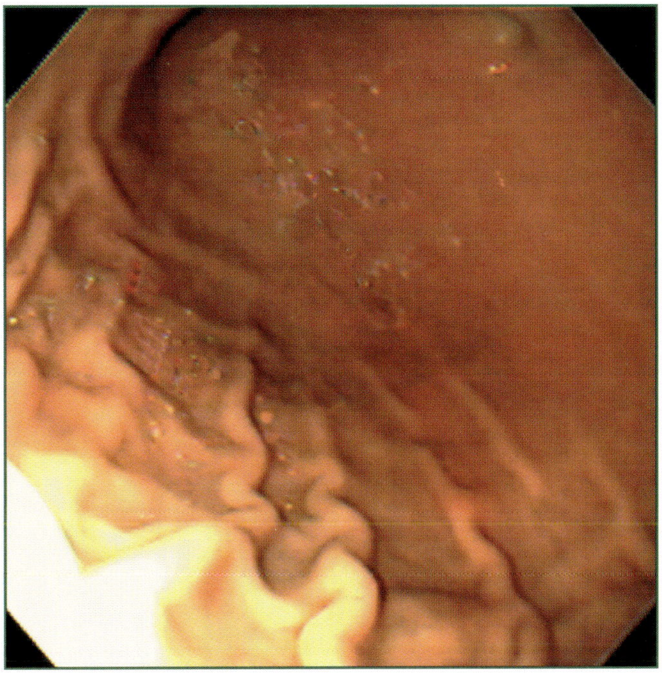

Figure 3.7 **An endoscopic view of the stomach of a dog showing the greater curvature with gastric rugae.**

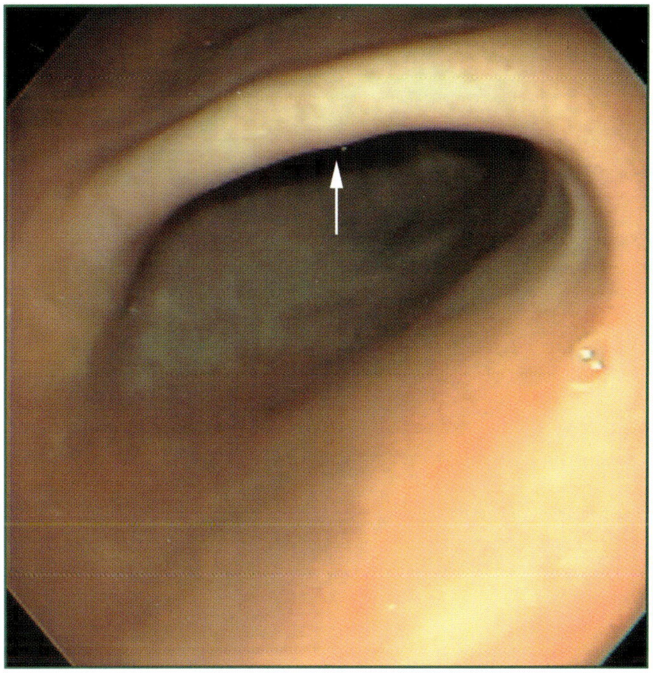

Figure 3.8 **An endoscopic view of the canine antrum showing the gastric angle (arrow), which is the demarcation between the lesser curvature and antrum.**

promise, causes ischemic-associated mucosal color changes, and also makes endoscopic entry through the pylorus more difficult. As the endoscope is advanced, by following the direction of the gastric rugae in the greater curvature, it progresses to the antrum. At the level of the antral opening is the incisura angularis (or gastric angle), which appears as a fold of tissue across the distal end of the body of the stomach when the stomach is inflated (***Figure 3.8***). This is an important anatomic landmark that divides the lesser curvature of the stomach from the antrum.

The distal tip of the endoscope can then either be advanced into the antrum or placed in a retroversion position, or "J position," a maneuver that provides a view of the lesser curvature, cardia, and fundus of the stomach (***Figure 3.9***). When the endoscope is moved into the antrum, the pylorus becomes evident. The normal antrum of the stomach is generally devoid of gastric rugae, and the pyloric opening is located at the distal end of the antral canal (***Figure 3.10***).

Occasionally, difficulties occur in examining the stomach. Sometimes during advancement of the endoscope in the direction of the antrum, there is a paradoxical backing up of the scope as it moves forward. This paradoxical movement occurs because pressure from the endoscope insertion tube expands the stomach along the greater curvature and, thus, the distal tip backs up. This problem can

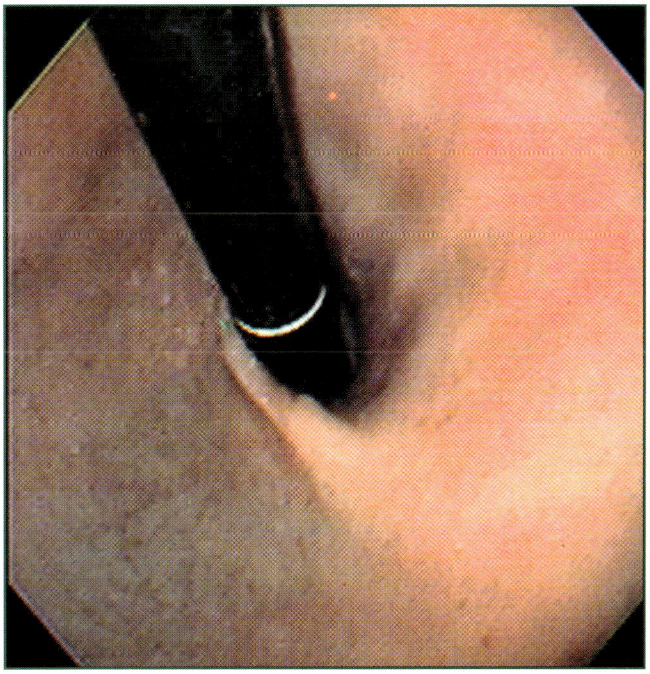

Figure 3.9 **An endoscopic view of the canine cardia. The endoscope is retroflexed using the "J maneuver" to see this region of the stomach.**

often be remedied simply by withdrawing the endoscope to just distal to the LES to decrease the lumen size, then readvancing the endoscope. Another problem that can often occur—again, when the stomach is overdistended with

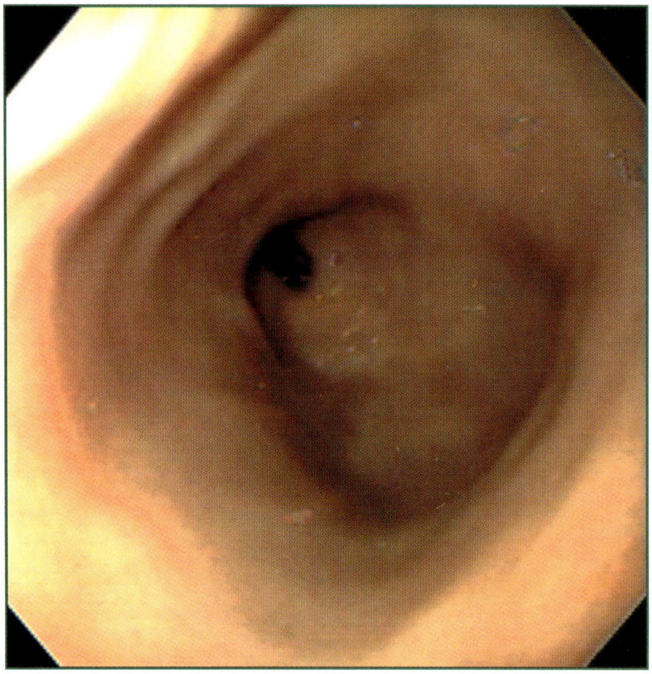

Figure 3.10 Endoscopic view of the canine pylorus.

air—is one in which the endoscope forms a full loop in the stomach making advancement more difficult than usual.

The normal gastric mucosa is smooth and has a pink to red color. Sometimes the appearance may be splotchy as the result of vascular changes from overinsufflation. Mucosal color changes are not always indicative of abnormalities. Endoscopic clues to gastric mucosal abnormalities include ulceration, mucosal irregularities, failure of gastric rugae to flatten, hyperemia, and mucosal friability. With suspected gastric lesions, multiple biopsy samples should be obtained from the mucosa. The biopsy forceps should be directed perpendicular to the mucosa using a pinch-and-pull technique. Because mucosal lesions may be regional in location, representative specimens should be taken from the fundus, greater and lesser curvature, and antrum. Mucosal brush cytology as well as fluid analysis may also be helpful and should be considered in all cases. In patients with gastric ulceration, luminal gastric pH should be determined by placing a drop of fluid on pH paper. Identifying very acidic gastric pH (approximately pH 1) could be a clue to hypergastric acid secretion from a gastrinoma or histamine release from mastocytosis. Biopsy specimens for *Helicobacter* spp culture are placed in urea broth or slant culture tubes and should also be obtained in animals with gastric disease.

Gastric Abnormalities

Foreign Bodies

Gastric foreign bodies are common and many can be removed using an endoscope in combination with various kinds of grasping forceps, snares, or baskets. The limiting factors of foreign-body removal are the ability to grasp the foreign body and the ability to withdraw the object through the LES.

Before induction of anesthesia for endoscopic removal, the current position of the foreign material should be confirmed radiographically. Often foreign bodies move between the time of making the diagnosis and performing the endoscopy. With the animal in left lateral recumbency, most freely movable foreign bodies are located in the fundic region of the stomach just inside and ventral to the LES. Sometimes foreign bodies located in this area are best viewed when the endoscope is placed in a retroflexed or J position, which is used to view the cardia and fundic region. If the foreign body is not readily apparent on endoscopic examination, placing the animal in different positions may help in locating the object. The presence of fluid and food in the stomach makes identification much more difficult. If there is considerable food in the stomach, it may be advisable to wait for the stomach to empty before endoscopy. However, this decision is made only if the delay will not compromise the animal.

After the foreign body is identified with the endoscope, it is firmly grasped with the appropriate retrieval forceps, basket, or snare (***Figure 3.11***). A large smooth object, such as a rock, is best removed using a basket; while a smaller object having an edge, such as a coin, can be grasped and removed with a forceps (***Figure 3.12***). When the foreign body is adequately secured with the retrieval instrument, both the endoscope and grasper are retracted together slowly.

Problems frequently occur when attempting to retract an object through the LES. It is at this point in the procedure that large objects often drop off the grasper and fall back into the stomach. To prevent loss of the object as it is withdrawn through the LES, the distal tip of the endoscope should be angled parallel to the lumen of the LES and slowly withdrawn through the sphincter with gradually increasing pressure. When difficulties arise while pulling the foreign object through the LES, it may be necessary to place a large-bore stomach tube over the endoscope and through the LES. This enables the endoscopist to pull the foreign body into the large stomach tube that distends the LES and remove both the tube and the endoscope as a unit

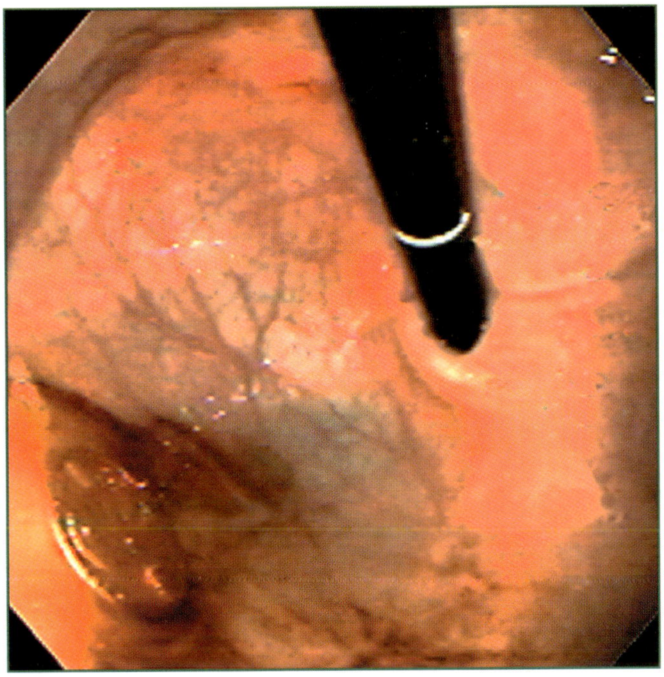

Figure 3.11 A penny foreign body in the fundic region of the stomach of a dog. This patient had developed zinc toxicity from the penny.

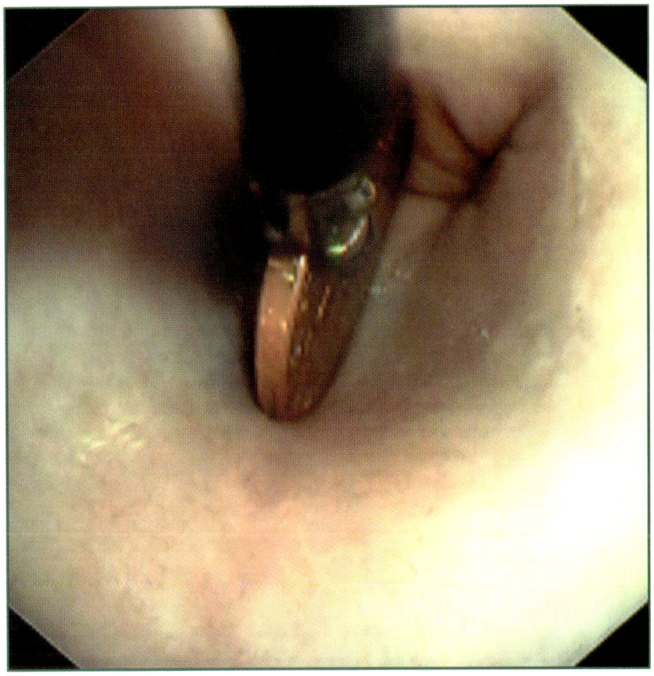

Figure 3.12 The penny foreign body shown in *Figure 3.11* being removed with grasping forceps. The location is in the distal esophagus.

(***Figure 3.13***). Also available are specially designed hoods that can be placed over the distal end of the endoscope to aid in foreign-body removal.

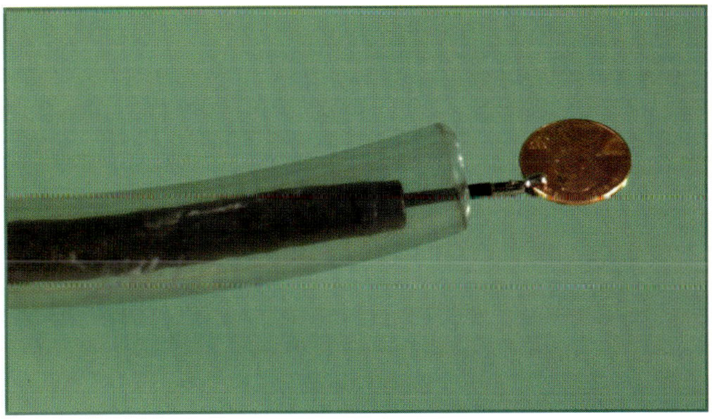

Figure 3.13 An example of a large-bore tube placed over the endoscope for foreign body removal. Pulling the foreign body to the tip of the tube or into the tube may aid in removal of large objects through the lower esophageal sphincter and esophagus.

Gastritis

Gastric mucosal inflammation is common; however, the etiology of many cases may never be determined. Such factors as chemicals, dietary substances (food allergies or intolerance), and drugs are all possible causes. Infectious causes, such as fungal, bacterial, and parasitic agents, are also factors to be considered in the etiology of gastritis. A spiral bacterium, *Helicobacter* sp, has been identified in the stomachs of dogs and cats with chronic lymphocytic-plasmacytic gastritis. The incidence and clinical significance of this organism causing chronic gastritis is still under investigation.

The endoscopic appearance of gastritis is highly variable. In some cases, the mucosa may look endoscopically normal but there is evidence of disease on histology. Consequently, biopsies should be done in all patients suspected of having gastric disease. Endoscopic clues to gastritis include mucosal friability, mucosal irregularity, prominent lymphoid follicles, or gastric rugae that fail to flatten with gastric insufflation. Because of the friability of the mucosa, often much larger biopsy samples are retrieved as compared with samples taken from normal mucosa. Mucosal color change does not always reflect mucosal disease and is most often the result of vascular changes. Small mucosal erosions with hemorrhage may also be observed (***Figure 3.14***). *Helicobacter* sp-associated gastritis is characterized by prominent lymphoid follicles and, rarely, mucosal ulceration. Hypertrophic gastritis is associated with regional, large gastric rugae that persist even with gastric insufflation, while atrophic gastritis is associated with a thinner than normal mucosa characterized by visible submucosal blood vessels.

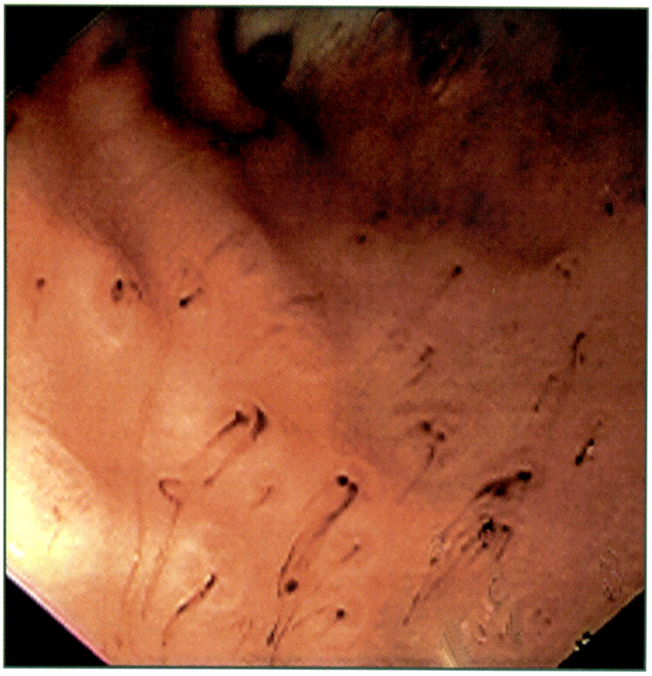

Figure 3.14 Small punctate erosions with hemorrhage in the stomach of a dog.

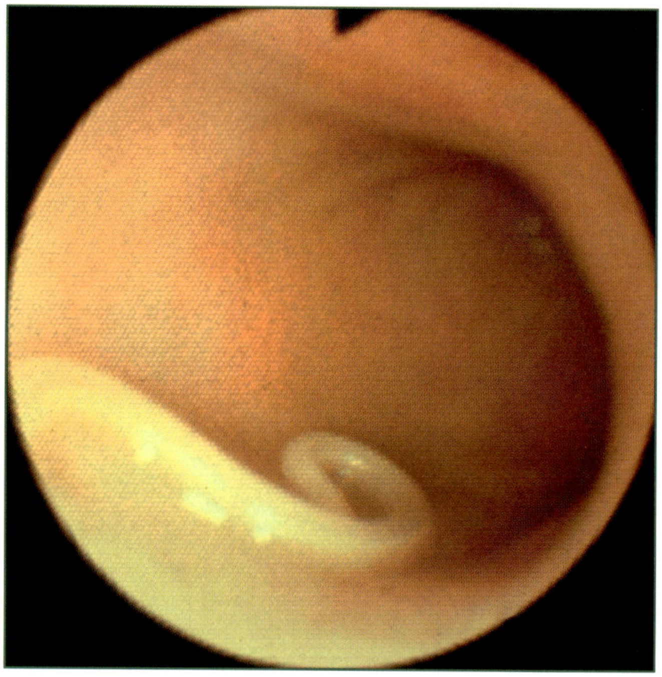

Figure 3.15 An ascarid in the duodenum of a cat.

Parasites

Gastric parasites are sometimes identified endoscopically (***Figure 3.15***). *Ollulanus tricuspis* is a small gastric parasite found in cats. The diagnosis of *Ollulanus tricuspis* infection is made by examining gastric fluid under a microscope on low power and looking for microfilariae resembling nematode parasites approximately 0.75 mm in length. Gastric fluid samples for examination can be collected during endoscopy. A second gastric parasite, *Physaloptera* sp, is also found in the stomach as well as the proximal duodenum in dogs and cats. *Physaloptera* sp is a cause of chronic vomiting but is difficult to diagnose because, on fecal examination, it is extremely uncommon to observe the parasite eggs in affected animals. The diagnosis is most frequently made during endoscopy by viewing the parasite in the stomach or proximal duodenum.

Gastric Ulceration

Ulceration refers to grossly detectable defects in the gastric mucosa. Most gastric ulcers usually appear as multiple, small, superficial mucosal erosions (*Figure 3.14*). It is uncommon to observe the conceptually typical ulcer characterized as a single, large "moon crater" ulcer. Animals with gastric ulceration usually also have blood in the gastric fluid. Blood may appear fresh, bright red or show a "coffee-ground" consistency, having undergone acid digestion. When gastric ulcers are observed, biopsy specimens should be taken from the ulcer as well as adjacent more normal-looking tissue. In performing a biopsy of a large ulcer, it is important to obtain tissue at the margin of the ulcer rather than at the center. Biopsy specimens taken from the center of an ulcer crater generally contain only necrotic tissue. Differentials for gastric mucosal ulceration are numerous but should include causes of gastric acid hypersecretion and neoplasia.

Pyloric Mucosal Antral Hypertrophy

Pyloric mucosal antral hypertrophy is a condition characterized by gastric mucosal hypertrophy in the antral and pyloric region of the stomach resulting in obstruction of gastric outflow. The condition is most often observed in small middle-aged or older dogs. Signs are chronic vomiting of food or gastric secretions.

The radiographic diagnosis is made by identifying gastric retention on a barium contrast study resulting from large mucosal folds that obstruct gastric outflow, located in the antral region of the stomach. Endoscopically, they often appear as polypoid or large folds of mucosa proximal to the pyloric canal. Normally, the antral region of the stomach is devoid of gastric rugae; and, generally, biopsy of the tissue demonstrates normal mucosa.

Gastric Neoplasia

Several types of neoplasia occur in the stomach of dogs and cats. Benign tumors include mucosal polyps and leiomyomas that are often an incidental finding unless they obstruct gastric emptying. Gastric leiomyomas occur as smooth submucosal masses, frequently located in the cardiac region of the stomach. Often, if the endoscopist grabs the mucosa overlying the leiomyoma with a biopsy forceps, the mucosa will freely slide over the mass, indicating it is not firmly attached to superficial tissues. Leiomyomas generally do not cause problems unless ulceration or mechanical obstruction occurs because of their location.

Gastric lymphosarcoma is more common in cats than dogs and arises as a large mass-type lesion, most often in the body of the stomach. Ulceration may be present. Occasionally, a diffuse lymphosarcoma can appear as prominent gastric rugae that fail to flatten as the stomach is distended (***Figure 3.16***). Gastric adenocarcinoma is the most common malignant neoplasm in dogs. Location in order of frequency is pyloric-antrum, lesser curvature, then greater curvature.

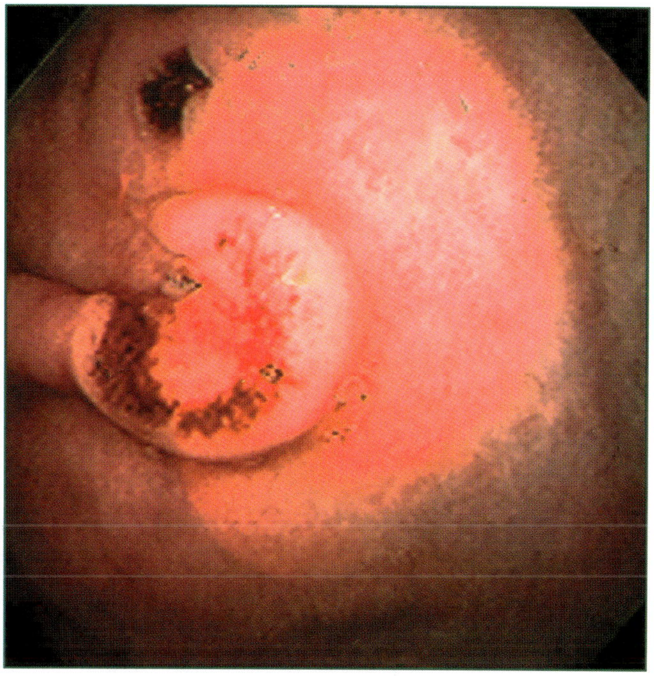

Figure 3.16 Endoscopic view of the stomach of a dog showing a large, ulcerated rugal fold. The gastric rugae failed to flatten as the stomach was insufflated. Biopsies confirmed gastric lymphoma.

Frequently, ulceration is present but some gastric adenocarcinomas may arise with only submucosal involvement. In these cases, the stomach becomes rigid and does not distend. Gastric rugae may also be large and prominent and do not flatten with insufflation of air. Mucosal ulceration can occur with gastric adenocarcinoma, however. Because of the typical submucosal involvement, superficial mucosal biopsies may not be diagnostic although deeper biopsies are positive. To obtain submucosal samples, one should repeat biopsies in the same spot, digging deeper into the tissue after each sample. If there is an ulcer present, samples should be taken at the margins and not in the center where there is only necrotic tissue. Other gastric neoplasms are reported in the stomach but they are less common.

Intestinal Endoscopy

Endoscopy of the small intestine has become an extremely valuable and minimally invasive means of obtaining intestinal biopsies. The procedure becomes very important in diagnosing various types of inflammatory bowel diseases and other intestinal mucosal disorders. Limitations of intestinal endoscopy, or enteroscopy, include both the difficulty that is sometimes encountered in passing the endoscope through the pylorus and the length of the endoscope insertion tube that can be advanced into the intestine. Most upper intestinal endoscopies are limited to the duodenum or the ileum when performing colonoscopy. A second limitation is the size of mucosal biopsy specimens that can be obtained by the biopsy forceps. In some situations, the biopsy samples may incorrectly represent the primary intestinal disease. This is especially true if the majority of the disease occurs in the submucosa or deeper layers. Nevertheless, gastrointestinal endoscopy is the least invasive means of performing an intestinal biopsy and is one of the most important diagnostic tools used in the evaluation of intestinal disease.

Indications

Indications for enteroscopy include signs of small intestinal disease, such as diarrhea, melena, and weight loss. Chronic vomiting is also an indication for endoscopic intestinal evaluation, because vomiting can be the predominant clinical sign in some cases of inflammatory bowel disease. Laboratory tests or imaging procedures that indicate intestinal disease are additional reasons for endoscopy.

Technique

Advancing the endoscope through the pylorus is the most difficult, and usually the most frustrating, aspect of gastrointestinal endoscopy. Pyloric entry requires considerable manipulative experience (and sometimes a little luck) to be successful. Upper intestinal endoscopy should be performed in all patients having gastroscopy. Duodenal entry is best achieved when the patient is placed in left lateral recumbency. After entering the stomach, the endoscope is quickly advanced through the stomach using minimal gastric distention to find the pylorus. Overdistention of the stomach with air or performing a complete gastric evaluation before attempting entry through the pylorus often makes the procedure more difficult.

After the scope has reached the pylorus, the endoscopist can identify the pyloric canal (*Figure 3.10*). The key to pyloric entry is to keep the pyloric canal centered in the middle of the endoscope's field of view as the instrument is slowly advanced. Slow, progressive movement forward while applying moderate, steady pressure to the endoscope tip should result in entry into the duodenum. With the endoscope centered in the pyloric canal, a small amount of insufflation often helps to open the lumen and aids in advancing the scope. When it is through the pyloric canal, the tip of the endoscope usually is in direct contact with the wall of the duodenum, obscuring the view and producing what is termed a "red-out." The lumen is not evident because of the sharp bend that occurs in the proximal duodenal bulb just beyond the pyloric canal. Manipulating the endoscope tip, generally down and to the right, with insufflation of a small amount of air usually identifies the duodenal lumen. The duodenal mucosa is whiter than the gastric mucosa and has a grainy appearance. A small amount of bile-colored fluid is often present in the lumen. When the lumen has been identified, the endoscope is then advanced as far as possible down the intestine.

Problems are commonly encountered in pyloric canal entry. Sometimes the pyloric opening is difficult to identify because it is obliterated by small gastric rugae. In these situations, it may be necessary to probe the area with a biopsy forceps to find the exact location of the pyloric opening. Another common problem occurs when the endoscope is not centered exactly in the pyloric canal and, consequently, the tip of the insertion tube contacts the antral wall and retroflexes back into the stomach when the endoscope is advanced.

After multiple unsuccessful attempts at pyloric entry, the endoscopist may elect to use the biopsy forceps as a guide to moving the endoscope's tip into the pylorus (***Figure 3.17***).

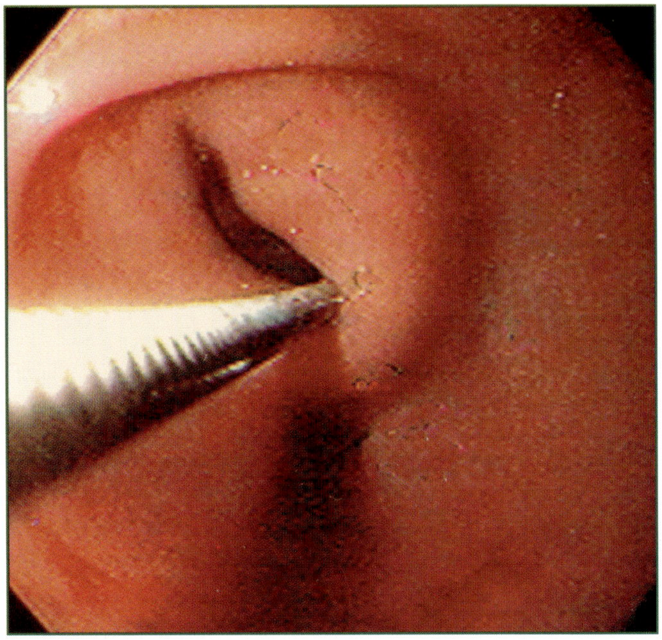

Figure 3.17 A biopsy forceps is shown here being used as a guide to help direct the endoscope tip through the pyloric canal of a dog.

To do this, the biopsy forceps is advanced 1 to 2 cm through the pyloric canal; and, by using careful endoscopic direction, the scope is then advanced into the duodenum. This technique results in generally minor, forceps-induced, superficial mucosal ulceration in the proximal duodenum. To date, no drugs have been proven to make endoscopic pyloric entry easier in the dog or cat. Some endoscopists prefer to avoid using atropine or narcotics as preanesthetic agents, suggesting that such avoidance facilitates pyloric entry; however, this recommendation is yet to be proved.

A normal duodenum appears reddish pink to whitish cream in color. The mucosa often has a velvety or shaggy appearance due to the intestinal villi. Following insufflation of the lumen, some of the granular texture will disappear. Peyer's patches or lymphoid nodules are identified in the descending duodenum as demarcated circular indentations that are within the mucosa but are paler in color (***Figure 3.18***). Often, Peyer's patches are referred to as "pseudo-ulcers." The endoscopist should also identify the duodenal papillae. In dogs, there are two: the proximal *major papilla* contains the common bile duct and is located on the medial wall 3 to 5 cm from the pylorus, with a *minor papilla*, containing the pancreatic ducts, on the dorsal wall 2 to 3 cm caudal to the major papilla. Cats have only a single duodenal papilla, which contains the common channel that drains the common bile duct and pancreatic ducts.

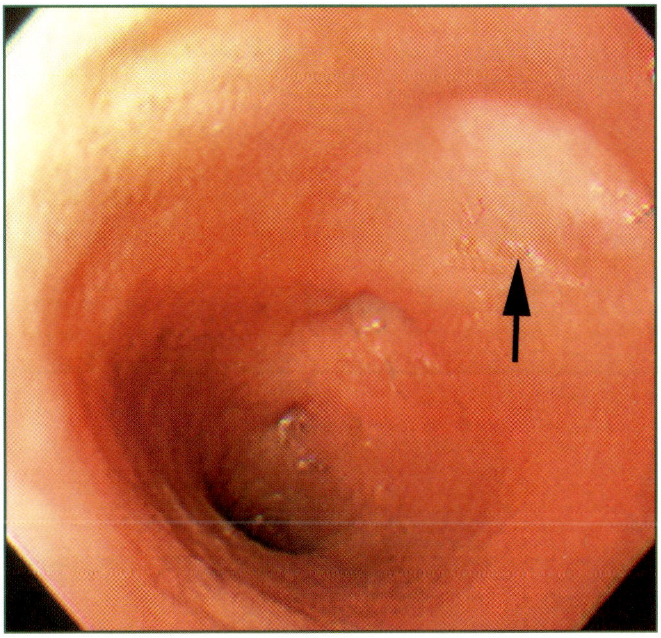

Figure 3.18 Endoscopic view of the normal canine duodenum showing Peyer's patches (arrow).

Frequently, in smaller animals, or with endoscopes having a long insertion tube, the jejunum can be reached.

Once the endoscope has been advanced as far as possible, which is dictated primarily by the endoscope insertion tube length, mucosal biopsy specimens are taken as the endoscope is withdrawn. There are two methods of performing small intestinal biopsies. The first is the blind technique, which involves advancing the forceps until resistance is felt. This usually occurs at the junction of the descending and ascending duodenum. The forceps is withdrawn a short distance, opened, and then advanced to the mucosa, where a sample is obtained. A second biopsy technique is visually directed. The area to be biopsied is determined, the endoscope tip is angled to the wall as perpendicularly as possible, and the forceps is advanced to the mucosa and a sample taken. This technique often results in the forceps sliding down the mucosa because the angle of direction is too closely parallel to the intestinal wall. Frequently, use of a biopsy forceps with a central needle, or "spike," prevents this problem from occurring. To aid either biopsy technique, it is advisable to deflate the lumen somewhat to reduce luminal tension, making it easier to grasp the mucosa. Intestinal biopsy usually causes minimal bleeding.

Fluid aspiration and brush cytology can also be performed during endoscopy. Additional samples can be taken using biopsy brushes or aspiration tubes for cytologic analysis. Cytology samples are inspected for inflammatory cells, parasites, or neoplasia. Fluid samples taken from the proximal duodenum can be quantitatively cultured to determine total bacterial numbers, indicating whether there is bacterial overgrowth (see the discussion on page 26).

Intestinal Abnormalities

Changes in mucosal texture are associated most frequently with histologic abnormalities; however, changes in mucosal color do not always predict mucosal disease. In either case, histologic assessment is always necessary. There seems to be considerable discord between the endoscopic appearance and the histologic interpretation of mucosal biopsy specimens.

Parasites

Giardia spp are flagellate protozoa that can cause acute and chronic diarrhea in dogs and cats. Diagnosis requires fecal tests by smear, flotation, or ELISA. The diagnosis can also be made during intestinal biopsy by observing the organism histologically on the mucosal surface or through duodenal fluid aspiration and microscopic cytologic evaluation. Duodenal fluid aspiration and cytology can be an accurate means of diagnosing *Giardia* organisms in the dog because they colonize in the proximal gastrointestinal tract; but, in cats, *Giardia* spp colonize in the distal small intestine. Because *Giardia* spp are a possible cause of gastrointestinal disease, endoscopic samples should be collected for analysis in appropriate cases. Other parasites that may be observed in the duodenum include *Physaloptera* spp and ascarids.

Idiopathic Inflammatory Bowel Disease

Idiopathic inflammatory bowel disease (IBD) is usually classified on the basis of the type of inflammatory cell infiltration that is present in the mucosa and, often, deeper layers. In fact, there is considerable confusion and controversy over this disease syndrome; and it has been stated that the ability to interpret biopsy specimens lags far behind the ability to obtain them. The endoscopic appearance of IBD is quite variable. It is reported that, in up to 65% of IBD cases, patients may have normal intestinal mucosa when viewed endoscopically. Endoscopic findings suggesting IBD include irregular mucosa, nodularity, and color changes (***Figure 3.19***). Also, subjectively, IBD patients generally provide larger mucosal biopsy samples than are

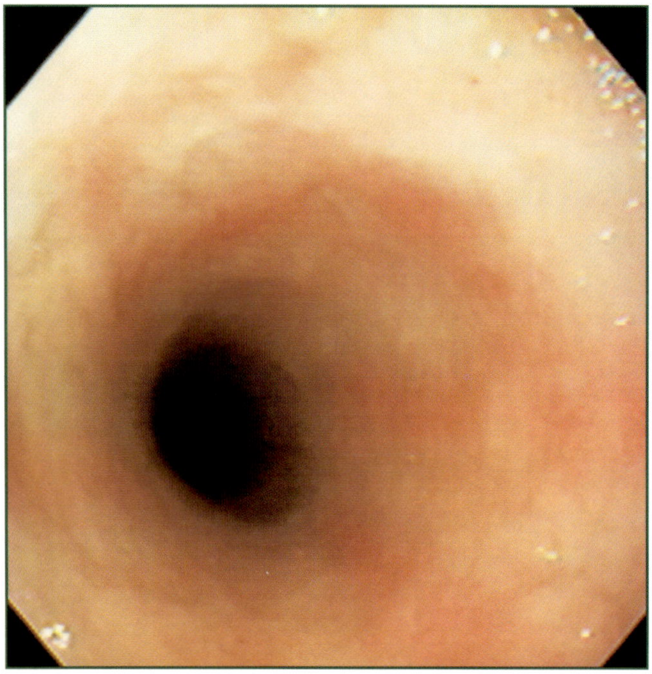

Figure 3.19 Endoscopic view of the duodenum of a dog with inflammatory bowel disease. The mucosa has an irregular surface and is hyperemic.

obtained from normal mucosa because of the increased friability. *These findings, however, are nonspecific and do not reflect the severity of disease.*

Granulomatous enteritis is an uncommon inflammatory intestinal disease characterized by inflammation with aggregates of histiocytes in the lamina propria. This condition is seen in both the dog and cat. When viewed endoscopically, the mucosa is almost always irregular and has a granular surface, often with ulceration. The lesion is generally segmental—involving the ileum, colon, or rectum by the granulomatous process—and results in luminal narrowing, mucosal ulceration, and mucosal rigidity. Practically speaking, it appears much like an intestinal neoplasm.

Bacterial Overgrowth

Bacterial overgrowth is a poorly understood condition that occurs in both dogs and cats. The regulation of bacterial numbers depends on many factors, including gastric acid secretion, intestinal secretions, local immunity, motility, and diet. Consequently, there are a number of potential conditions that could result in increased microflora and subsequent clinical signs. Bacterial overgrowth may arise from a primary motility disorder, a partial obstruction, reduced gastric acid production, or exocrine pancreatic insufficiency; or it may be idiopathic.

There are several tests available that support the diagnosis of small intestinal bacterial overgrowth. The so-called "gold standard" for the diagnosis is quantitation of bacterial numbers in the proximal small intestine after an 8-hour fast. In dogs, finding greater than 10^5 colony-forming units per milliliter of duodenal fluid is considered abnormal. Cats have higher numbers of colony-forming bacteria, with concentrations of 10^8 found in normal animals. Consequently, culturing duodenal juice using endoscopic aspiration through sterile tubing confirms the diagnosis. Care should be taken to prevent oral contamination and dilution of duodenal fluid with the water flush that is used for cleaning the endoscope lens. Also, animals that receive atropine during anesthesia frequently produce less gastrointestinal secretions, making it more difficult to recover fluid.

Lymphangiectasia

Lymphangiectasia is a common disorder of unknown etiology associated with marked dilatation of the intestinal mucosal and submucosal lymphatics. It is reported to be the most common cause of a protein-losing enteropathy. Impaired intestinal drainage caused by obstruction to normal lymph flow leads to stasis of chyle in the dilated lacteals and lymphatics of the bowel wall and mesentery. The distended lacteals then leak lymph (protein, fat, and lymphocytes) into the intestinal lumen, resulting in panhypoproteinemia, lymphopenia, hypocholesterolemia, and fat malabsorption.

The diagnosis requires excluding all other causes of low proteins. IBD, intestinal lymphosarcoma, and histoplasmosis are just a few examples of intestinal protein-losing enteropathies. Endoscopically, the villi appear dilated because of the prominent lacteals, which are characterized by white villous tips. The mucosa may take on a white, lacy appearance. Sometimes feeding a small amount of fat several hours before the endoscopy will make the villi stand out.

Intestinal Neoplasia

Neoplastic lesions are sometimes observed in the proximal small intestine or during colonoscopy in the ileum. Intestinal lymphoma may be either a diffuse infiltration or a regional mass. In cases of diffuse intestinal lymphoma, the mucosa may appear normal or may be irregular in appearance, similar to IBD. Focal neoplastic lesions, such as lymphoma, adenocarcinoma, leiomyoma, or even mucosal polyps, often result in mucosal ulceration, narrowing of the luminal diameter, and mucosal irregularity. There may be evidence of gastrointestinal bleeding or intestinal obstruction with some focal lesions.

Other Findings

Conditions sometimes observed during intestinal endoscopy include intestinal foreign bodies, intussusception, fungal disease, and duodenal ulceration. Although an uncommon finding, duodenal ulceration may occur from conditions resulting in increased gastric acid production or from nonsteroidal anti-inflammatory drug therapy.

Colonoscopy

Colonoscopy is the technique for examination of the rectum and large intestine. It can be performed using either a rigid hollow proctoscope or flexible gastrointestinal endoscope. A rigid proctoscope limits the examination to the rectum and the descending colon; while the flexible gastrointestinal endoscope allows examination of the entire colon, cecum, and, frequently, the ileum.

Indications

Generally, colonoscopy is performed in animals showing chronic signs of large bowel diarrhea. These signs include tenesmus, urgency, frequency, and/or dyschezia. Stool containing mucus or fresh blood also suggests colonic disease. In addition, colonoscopy with colonic biopsies should be considered for animals with signs of small intestinal disease. This is because distal small intestinal disorders may not be detected in some patients by upper gastrointestinal endoscopy but are identified through colonoscopy because of concurrent large intestinal involvement.

A complete laboratory evaluation is indicated prior to endoscopic examination and should include a fecal examination for parasites. Fecal cytology, mucosal scrapings, and cytology or fecal cultures may also provide diagnostic information that could preclude the need for endoscopy. Imaging studies, such as ultrasound and radiographic barium contrast enemas, generally offer less useful information when flexible colonoscopy is available. Colonoscopy should not be performed in patients with acute bacterial colitis or patients that have had recent colonic surgery.

Technique

The key to successful colonoscopy is adequate patient preparation. Many protocols are described for colonoscopy, and most are time and management intensive; but it is essential to assure that the colon is free of fecal material. ***Table 3.1*** highlights one technique used for colonic preparation in dogs. Two keys to success are withholding solid food for at least 36 to 48 hours and administering multiple warm-water enemas over that time period. Some techniques also involve concurrent oral administration of a gastrointestinal lavage solution, typically via a gastric tube. These cathartic lavage solutions, when given to reach to a large total volume, result in osmotic diarrhea and are quite successful in cleansing the large intestine. Gastrointestinal lavage solutions are safe and do not cause significant electrolyte abnormalities or dehydration.

Cats are generally much easier to prepare for colonoscopy because of their proportionally smaller and simpler colon. In most cases, fasting and multiple warm-water enemas are adequate and negate the need for lavage solutions. Soaps should not be added to the enema fluid as they may result in mucosal hyperemia. Generally, warm water is all that is required. Phosphate enemas should be avoided because of toxicity.

Flexible fiberoptic colonoscopy should only be performed with the animal placed under general anesthesia. Narcotic agents should be avoided because they stimulate intestinal motility and may move small intestinal fluid into the colon. The animal should be placed in left lateral recumbency so that the ileum, cecum, and ascending colon are in a superior position, which simplifies examination of the area. A digital rectal examination should always be performed before endoscopy to rule out rectal lesions or a diverticulum.

TABLE 3.1 SUGGESTED COLONIC PREPARATION TECHNIQUE FOR DOGS

Preparation Period	*Procedure*
36-48 hr before procedure	Withhold solid food
24 hr before procedure	1st warm-water enema Gastrointestinal lavage* (30 ml/kg body weight; 2 doses orally 2-4 hr apart) 2nd warm-water enema
Day of procedure	3rd warm-water enema Perform colonoscopy

* GoLYTELY, NuLYTELY—Braintree Laboratories, Braintree, MA.

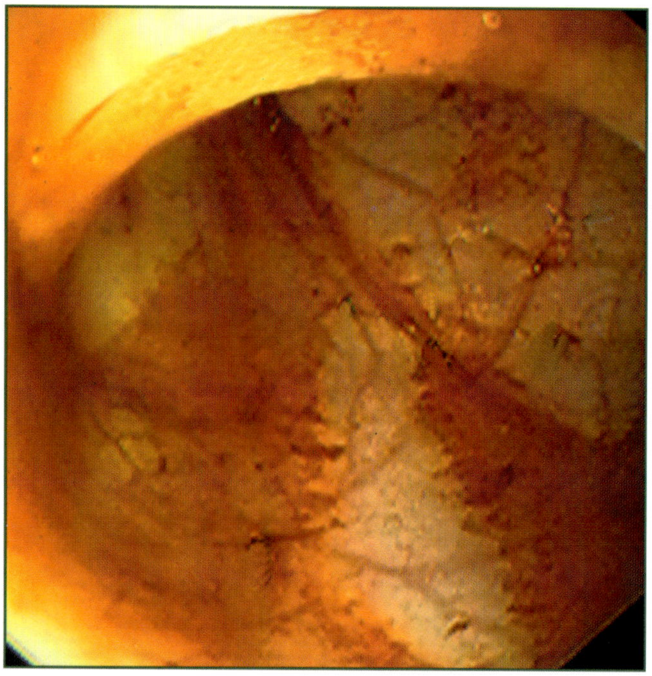

Figure 3.20 A close-up endoscopic view of the normal canine colon showing submucosal blood vessels. Mucus and residual fecal material is seen over the surface of the mucosa.

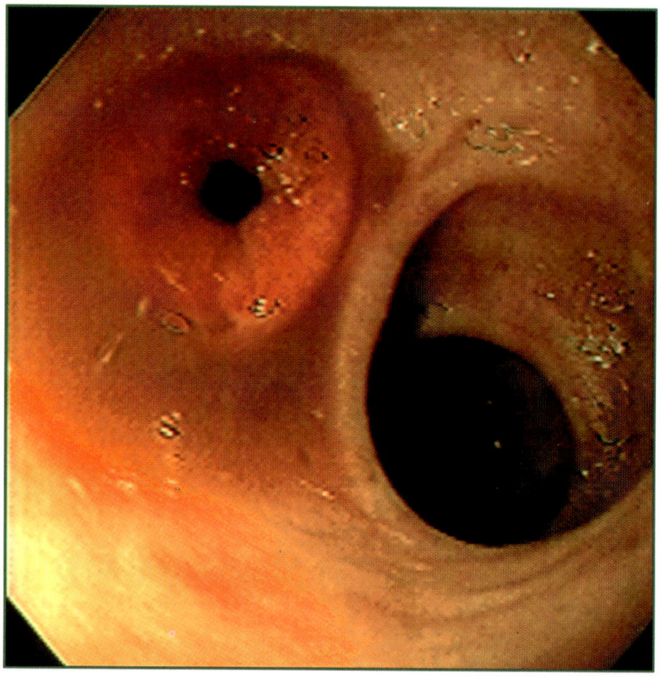

Figure 3.21 An endoscopic view of the normal canine proximal ascending colon showing the larger opening into the cecum and the smaller ileocolic sphincter opening.

The endoscope is first advanced through the anus and into the rectum. The colon is insufflated with air; and, as the lumen is visualized, the endoscope is passed. A commonly encountered problem is air escaping around the anal sphincter during insufflation because of the decreased anal tone associated with general anesthesia. This often requires manually holding the sphincter closed around the endoscope insertion tube to prevent air loss. Residual fluid in the colon is also aspirated using the endoscope suction.

A normal colon has a smooth glistening surface, and the submucosal blood vessels can be seen (***Figure 3.20***). The mucosa should not be friable or bleed easily when touched by the endoscope. As the endoscope is advanced, the colon makes a number of turns that must be navigated. To advance the endoscope past the hepatic and splenic flexures, which are sharp right-angle turns demarcating the junction of the transverse colon, a slide-by technique is usually required. Because it becomes difficult to navigate the endoscope around these sharp corners, the endoscope must be blindly advanced along the wall of the colon around the turns. This is the one endoscopic situation in which the lumen cannot be observed during scope advancement.

The next landmark is the ileocecocolic junction. It is at this level that the opening of the cecum and the ileocolic sphincter are viewed (***Figure 3.21***). The cecum is quite large in dogs and sometimes may not be recognized as such by the endoscopist, who thinks he/she is still in the colon. Unknowingly in the cecum, the endoscopist quickly becomes "lost" and cannot find the lumen because the cecum is a blind-ended pouch. The ileocolic valve is adjacent to the cecal opening and appears as a thickened sphincter. In some cases, the endoscope can be directed through the ileocolic valve into the ileum. If entry into the ileum is not possible by scope, it may be feasible to carefully advance a biopsy forceps blindly into the ileum to collect mucosal samples.

At the completion of visual examination of the large intestine, the endoscope is slowly withdrawn and biopsy samples and/or brush cytology samples are then collected. Before withdrawing the scope from the rectum, it is retroflexed into a J position in such a manner as to view the distal rectum and anorectal junction (***Figure 3.22***).

Colonic Abnormalities

Table 3.2 lists common endoscopic abnormalities found in the large intestine. Evidence of abnormal colonic mucosa include findings similar to those described for the small intestine but also include failure of the lumen to distend when insufflated with air and the loss of the presence of the submucosal blood vessels. A definitive diagnosis is made through biopsy and histology.

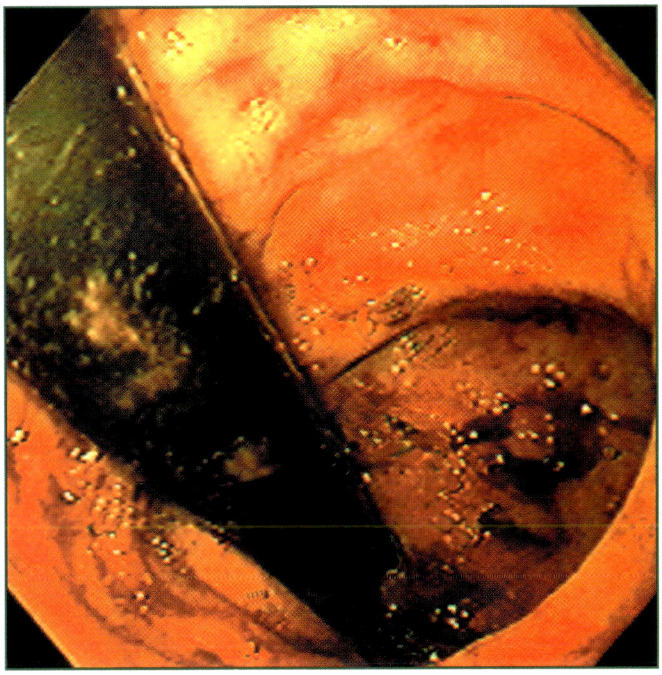

Figure 3.22 An endoscopic view of the rectum looking distally with the endoscopic tip placed in the "J position."

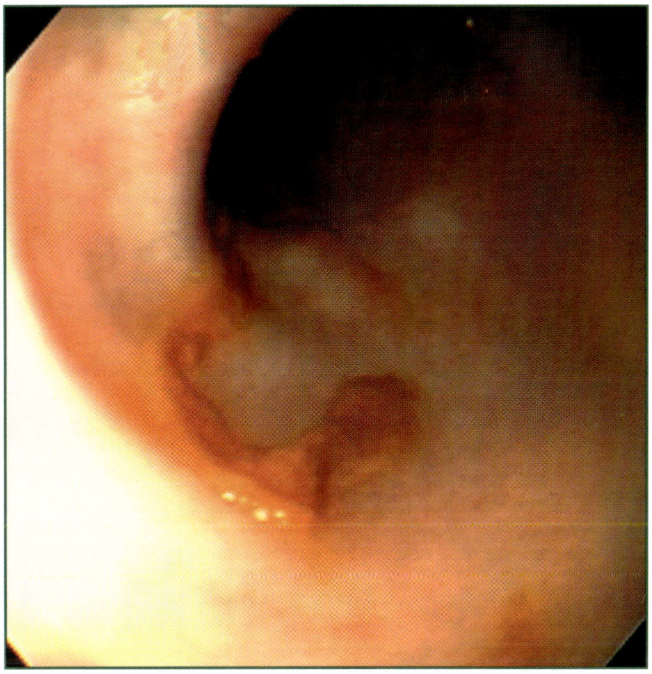

Figure 3.23 An endoscopic view of the descending colon in a cat with lymphocytic plasmacytic colitis. The submucosal blood vessels cannot be seen, which is suggestive of mucosal infiltration.

TABLE 3.2 COMMON FINDINGS IN THE COLON

- ❑ Cecal inversion
- ❑ Colitis
- ❑ Colonic ulceration
- ❑ Foreign bodies
- ❑ Fungal colitis
- ❑ Granulomatous lesions
- ❑ Ileocolic intussusception
- ❑ Neoplasia
- ❑ Parasites
- ❑ Polyps
- ❑ Strictures

Parasitic Colitis

Parasites are a common cause of colitis in the dog. Both hookworms and whipworms can infect the proximal colon and can be identified endoscopically while attached to the mucosa. An eosinophilic colitis is also often associated with intestinal parasites.

Idiopathic Chronic Colitis

Idiopathic chronic colitis or inflammatory bowel disease involving the colon is characterized by variable populations of inflammatory cells (lymphocytes, plasmacytes, neutrophils, or eosinophils) in the mucosal and deeper layers. The etiology of chronic colitis is unknown; but, in most cases, an intraluminal factor is suspected as the initiating agent. Dietary components, infectious agents, bacteria or their by-products, parasites, or possibly extension of immune-mediated mechanisms may be responsible. Eosinophilic colitis appears to be associated most often with parasitic or dietary factors. Typically, an etiologic agent is never determined and the inflammation is speculated to be due to a defect in colonic immunoregulation.

Endoscopic findings include hyperemia, increased mucosal granularity, friability, loss of submucosal blood vessels, lymphoid follicles, mucosal irregularity, and erosive changes (***Figure 3.23***). The mucosa may bleed easily when touched by the endoscope, while in the normal colon it is quite resistant to iatrogenic trauma. Generally, the descending colon is involved; but lesions may be regional or patchy, indicating the need for obtaining multiple, representative biopsy samples.

Granulomatous Colitis

Granulomatous colitis is usually regional, involving the distal small intestine and/or colon. The condition is typically associated with a transmucosal chronic inflammatory disease, and its clinical appearance is often similar to that of neoplastic lesions. Histolytic ulcerative colitis of boxer dogs and fungal colitis (histoplasmosis) also appear similar to granulomatous colitis endoscopically. Findings include mucosal irregularity, variable degree of ulceration and hemorrhage, and decreased wall distensibility. Lesions may result in a narrowing or stricture of the colon. Multiple, deep biopsies are required to make the diagnosis.

Cecal Inversion

Cecal inversion or cecocolonic invagination and ileocolic intussusceptions are uncommon disorders. Cecal inversions result in invagination of the cecum into the lumen of the colon causing partial obstruction. They occur most often in conjunction with whipworm infections. The inversions appear as small fingerlike projections of normal-looking mucosa in the lumen. By contrast, ileocolic intussusceptions occur as larger, smooth intraluminal masses generally causing almost complete obstruction of the colonic lumen. Biopsy of either kind of lesion usually returns as normal epithelium.

Colonic Polyps

Colonic polyps typically occur in the distal colon. Because of their distal location, identification may require retroflexing the endoscope in a caudal direction for viewing. Polyps are single or multiple, with either a pedunculate stalk or a sessile base. Biopsy is often unreliable because only superficial mucosa is obtained. Treatment involves surgical excision or an endoscopic snare-loop polypectomy. Some polyps may transform to carcinoma in situ or to malignant neoplasia.

Colonic Neoplasia

Colonic neoplasia is uncommon in dogs and cats. Clinical signs usually include hematochezia, dyschezia, tenesmus, and mucoid diarrhea. Benign tumors include adenomas and leiomyomas. The most common malignant tumors are lymphosarcoma and adenocarcinoma. Most arise in the descending colon and rectum. Adenocarcinomas generally appear similar to granulomatous colitis, with obstruction of the colonic lumen (***Figure 3.24***). Lymphosarcoma may arise as a single mass lesion or as a diffuse involvement. Deep biopsy is required for a diagnosis of colonic neoplasia. This is accomplished by repeated sampling at the same site to obtain deeper submucosal tissue.

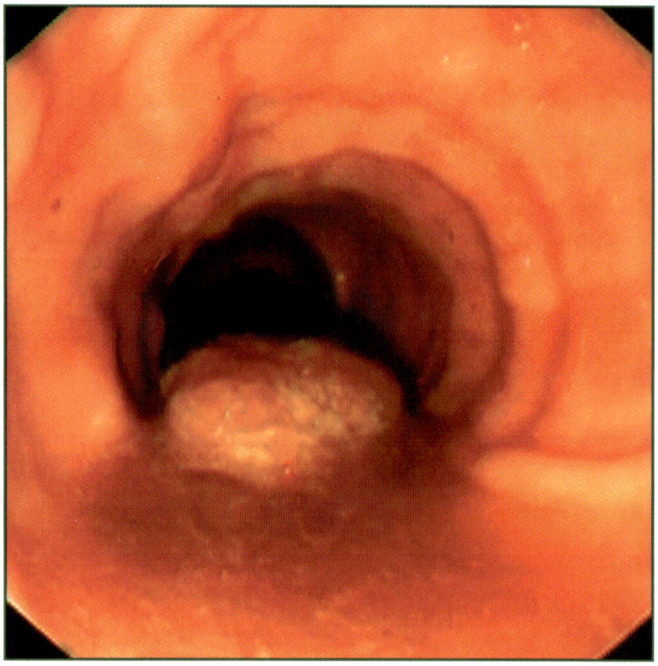

Figure 3.24 An endoscopic view of a mass located in the descending colon of a dog. Biopsy of the mass revealed colonic adenocarcinoma.

Chapter 4: **Case Studies**

CASE 1

SIGNALMENT: 4-year-old spayed female Siamese cat

HISTORY: There was a recent diagnosis of upper respiratory infection that was treated with doxycycline for 1 week. The owner reported that the respiratory signs had resolved; however, following recovery from the upper respiratory infection, the cat began progressive regurgitation. The cat was able to drink and keep down water but regurgitated solid food almost immediately after eating. The cat's appetite was good, and it often reingested the regurgitated food.

P.E.: The cat was thin but no other specific abnormalities were identified.

ENDOSCOPIC FINDINGS: A view of the esophageal lumen at the level of the thoracic inlet showed a 2-mm-diameter narrowing (*Figure 4.1*).

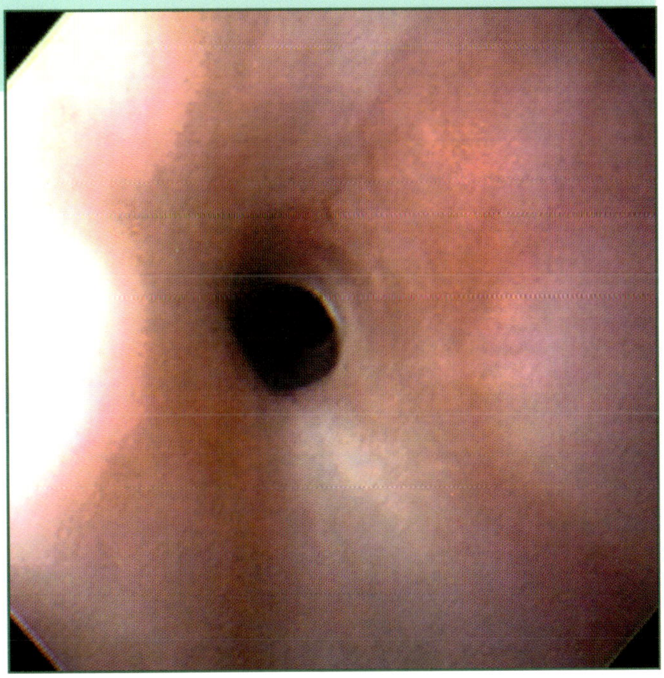

Figure 4.1 Esophageal stricture at the thoracic inlet in a cat.

Initial Assessment

This cat presented for regurgitation that suggested esophageal disease. The ability to hold down liquids combined with the inability to hold down solid food supports an esophageal obstruction. Causes for esophageal obstruction in an adult cat include a foreign body, stricture, tumor, or extra-esophageal mass compressing the esophagus.

Presumptive Diagnosis

Esophageal obstruction.

Diagnostic Plan

The esophagus was first evaluated by routine cervical and thoracic radiographs, which were normal. A barium contrast study was performed, initially using barium liquid, and no abnormalities were noted. However, a second esophagram using a food-barium mixture showed narrowing of the esophageal lumen at the thoracic inlet (*Figure 4.2*). The diagnosis of an esophageal stricture was made. Endoscopy confirmed the esophageal stricture with a concentric luminal narrowing to approximately 2 mm.

Outcome

The focal esophageal stricture was treated using balloon dilation (*Figure 4.3*). Balloon catheters of increasing diame-

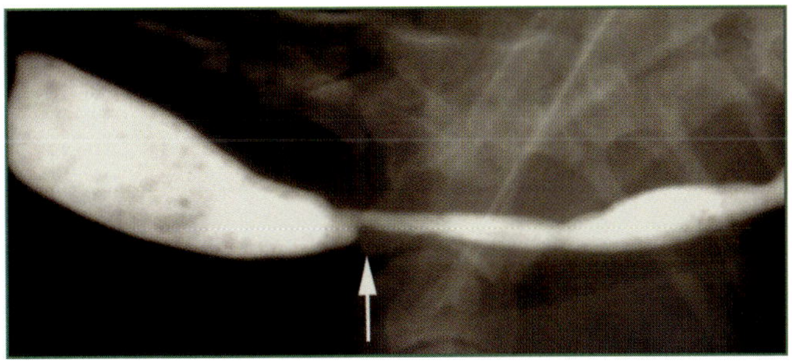

Figure 4.2 Using a food-barium mixture, an esophagram demonstrates luminal narrowing (arrow) at the thoracic inlet of a cat.

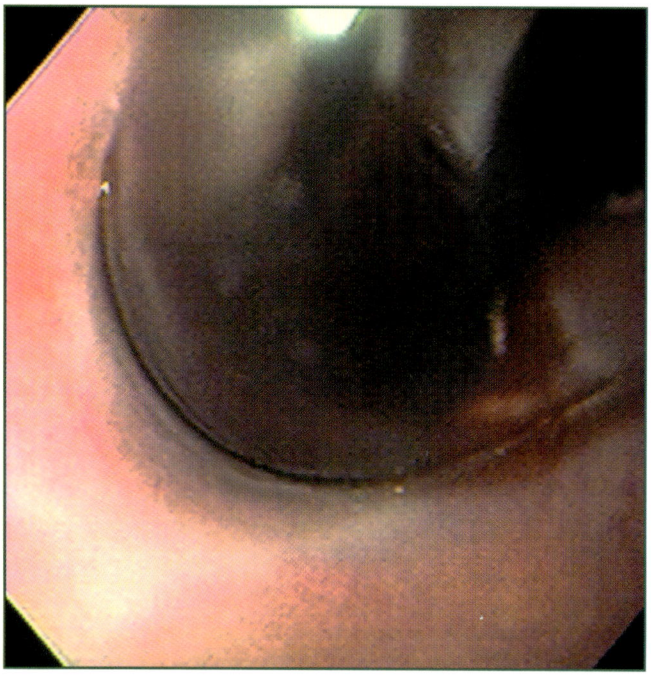

Figure 4.3 Endoscopic view of an inflated balloon dilator placed in the esophageal stricture.

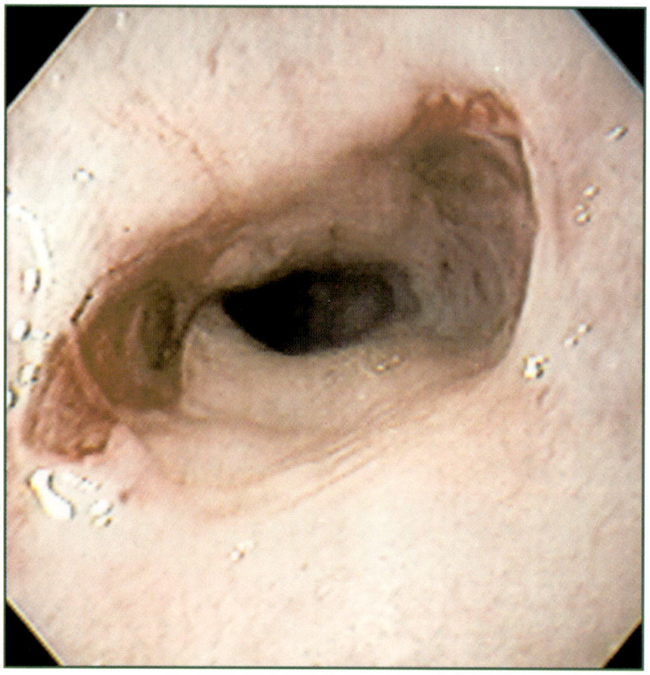

Figure 4.4 Endoscopic view of the strictured area in the esophagus (*Figure 4.1*) following balloon dilation.

ter were placed into the stricture and then slowly inflated under pressure. Using this technique, the esophageal lumen was dilated to an 18-mm diameter (*Figure 4.4*). The cat was treated with prednisolone to prevent refibrosis at the stricture site. Liquefied sucralfate was given orally for topical mucosal protection, omeprazole was given to block acid production, and cisapride was given to increase LES pressure to prevent gastric esophageal reflux.

Repeat dilations were performed at weekly intervals for a total of 3 treatments. The cat made an uneventful recovery and was able to hold down canned food without regurgitation.

Comment

Doxycycline tablets have been reported to cause esophageal strictures in cats, and the drug is suspected to be responsible for the stricture in this case. The caustic nature of this medication, along with failure of the pill to pass readily into the stomach, can result in a focal esophagitis and a subsequent fibrotic stricture.

Case 2

SIGNALMENT: 7-year-old castrated male Boston terrier dog

HISTORY: This dog had an 8-month history of regurgitation and/or vomiting that responded poorly to symptomatic therapy. The owner described relatively passive episodes of expulsion of gastric fluid and mucus that sometimes contained small amounts of food and occasionally was blood tinged. Episodes were intermittent, occurring up to several times a day. The dog's appetite was sporadic, and the owner complained that the dog had halitosis. This dog also had chronic brachycephalic respiratory complex, and surgery had previously been recommended.

P.E.: A significant inspiratory stridor was evident, with the corresponding elongated soft palate and stenotic nares. The remainder of the physical examination was unremarkable.

ENDOSCOPIC FINDINGS: An endoscopic view of the distal esophagus showed linear esophageal ulcerations with a small amount of food material in the lumen (*Figure 4.5*). The lower esophageal sphincter was open.

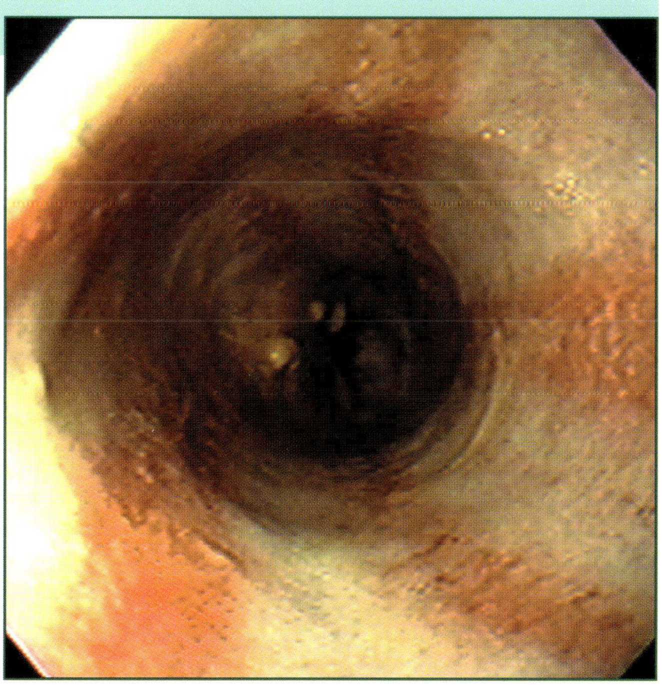

Figure 4.5 Endoscopic view of the distal esophagus showing linear esophageal ulcerations, refluxed gastric contents, and an open lower esophageal sphincter.

Initial Assessment

This dog presented with signs of chronic regurgitation, but it was uncertain whether vomiting was among the clinical signs. Blood present in the regurgitated fluid suggests mucosal ulceration. The differential diagnosis would include esophageal motility disorders, esophageal obstructive lesions, and inflammatory esophageal disease. Gastric disorders causing vomiting are less likely differentials because the owner did not report any active retching. The upper respiratory stridor was assumed to be associated with the dog's brachycephalic respiratory complex.

Presumptive Diagnosis

Inflammatory or ulcerative esophageal disease.

Diagnostic Plan

Routine thoracic and abdominal radiographs were taken to rule out obvious esophageal or gastric abnormalities and were normal. Results of a complete blood cell count (CBC), biochemical profile, and urinalysis obtained to evaluate for metabolic or systemic disease were within normal limits. A liquid barium esophagram was performed to evaluate esophageal function. There was abnormal delayed transit in the distal esophagus, suggesting inflammatory esophageal disease. Endoscopic examination of the esophagus showed linear mucosal ulcerations of the distal esophagus with a small amount of food and fluid in the lumen. The lower esophageal sphincter was open, suggesting gastroesophageal reflux as the cause of the esophagitis. The stomach was normal. Examination of the respiratory system identified stenotic nares, an elongated soft palate, and everted laryngeal saccules.

Outcome

This dog was treated for reflux esophagitis using liquefied sucralfate for topical mucosal protection, omeprazole to block gastric acid production, and metoclopramide to increase LES pressure and prevent acid reflux. The dog responded well to therapy, and its clinical signs resolved. After discontinuing the medication, clinical signs returned and the dog required further therapy. A subsequent surgery to correct the stenotic nares, elongated soft palate, and everted laryngeal saccules resolved all signs of the reflux esophagitis.

Comment

Reflux esophagitis is usually idiopathic but can also be secondary to the brachycephalic syndrome. It is suspected that the increased negative intrathoracic pressure in brachycephalic dogs can result in subsequent gastroesophageal reflux.

Case 3

SIGNALMENT: One-year-old female mixed-breed terrier dog

HISTORY: The dog was presented for acute onset of retching and regurgitation of 12 hours' duration. It was reluctant to eat but could hold down a small amount of water. The owner suspected the dog had something caught in its throat because it had gotten into garbage earlier the same day. The dog had been in good health prior to the current problem.

P.E.: The dog was lethargic and salivating. A complete oral examination was normal, and the remainder of the physical examination was unremarkable.

ENDOSCOPIC FINDINGS: An endoscopic view of the distal thoracic esophagus showed a bone foreign body (*Figure 4.6*).

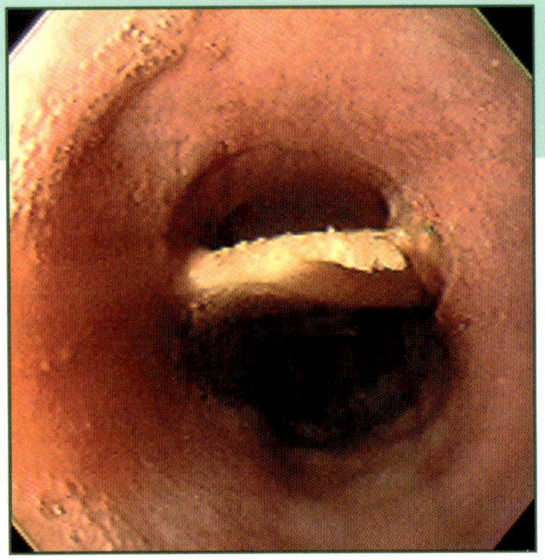

Figure 4.6 Endoscopic view of the distal esophagus with a bone foreign body.

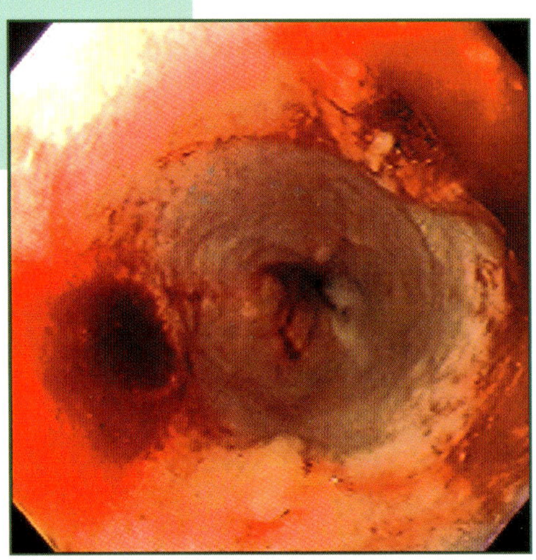

Figure 4.7 Endoscopic view of the esophagus following removal of a bone foreign body. Note the ulcerations in the esophageal wall where the bone was lodged.

Initial Assessment

Acute onset of retching and regurgitation with a history of garbage ingestion makes an esophageal foreign body causing esophageal obstruction a high-ranking differential in this case. Other differentials should include ingestion of caustic or abrasive substances causing esophagitis and ulceration.

Presumptive Diagnosis

Esophageal foreign body.

Diagnostic Plan

In cases of suspected esophageal foreign body, routine radiographs of the neck and thorax should be taken immediately. Routine films of this dog showed a small amount of gas in the esophagus with a bone density in the lumen of the esophagus proximal to the lower esophageal sphincter.

Endoscopy was performed, and a piece of a bone was found wedged in the lumen of the esophagus with each end embedded in the esophageal mucosa. The bone was removed using an endoscopic grasping forceps. Following removal of the bone, the esophagus was reexamined and two small mucosal ulcers were identified where the bone had eroded into the wall (*Figure 4.7*). The stomach was then evaluated for additional foreign material and was normal.

Outcome

The dog made an uneventful recovery. Because of the close proximity of the mucosal ulceration to the lower esophageal sphincter, the dog was treated for reflux esophagitis with famotidine to block gastric acid and cisapride to increase the lower esophageal sphincter pressure.

Comment

Bone esophageal foreign bodies most commonly lodge proximal to the lower esophageal sphincter and next most commonly at the level of the base of the heart. Large bones may require a rigid esophageal scope and a large, sturdy grasping forceps for removal. In cases of unsuccessful bone removal, the clinician should then attempt to push the bone into the stomach where it will undergo normal digestion.

Case 4

SIGNALMENT: Five-year-old castrated male Norwich terrier dog

HISTORY: Approximately 1 month before presentation, the dog had a bone esophageal foreign body just proximal to the lower esophageal sphincter. The bone was pushed into the stomach using endoscopic direction. Two small areas of mucosal ulceration were noted at the site of the bone foreign body. The dog was treated for esophagitis for 1 week and did well clinically. About 3 weeks later, the dog was presented again with the complaint of progressive increasing frequency of regurgitation of small amounts of fluid, mucus, and, occasionally, a little food. The regurgitation was not associated with eating, and the dog was able to consume normal meals. The dog was healthy in all other respects.

P.E.: No abnormalities were detected on physical examination.

ENDOSCOPIC FINDINGS: An endoscopic view of the distal esophagus and lower esophageal sphincter showed a large 1.2-cm opening in the lateral wall of the esophagus and an area of healing mucosa on the opposite side of the esophagus (*Figure 4.8*). The location of the defects was at the level of the previous esophageal foreign body.

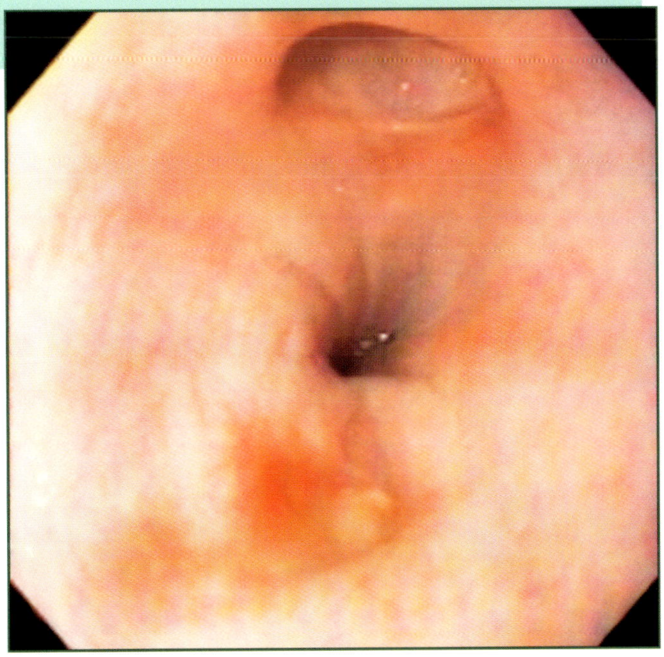

Figure 4.8 An endoscopic view of the distal esophagus and lower esophageal sphincter (LES). Dorsal to the LES is a 1.2-cm opening into a large diverticulum. Ventral to the LES is an area of ulceration from the previous bone foreign body.

Initial Assessment

The previous history of a bone esophageal foreign body with subsequent esophageal signs should suggest a post-foreign body removal problem. Differential diagnosis should include an esophageal motility defect, esophagitis, esophageal stricture formation, dysfunction of the lower esophageal sphincter, or an esophageal diverticulum. Because the dog was able to keep solid food down, an esophageal stricture was a less likely diagnosis in this case.

Presumptive Diagnosis

Functional or morphologic defect secondary to the previous bone foreign body.

Diagnostic Plan

Blood was submitted for a CBC, biochemical profile, and urinalysis. All laboratory tests were unremarkable. Routine thoracic radiographs were taken and showed increased density in the distal esophagus. A liquid barium contrast study was performed and showed delayed passage of the contrast medium through the distal esophagus, with marked barium retention in a 1 × 2-cm diverticulum at the level of the distal esophagus (*Figure 4.9*). Endoscopy confirmed an esophageal diverticulum just cranial to the lower esophageal sphincter. The endoscope tip could be directed through the mucosal defect into an approximately 2-cm diverticulum.

Outcome

Following endoscopy, the dog was taken to surgery for evaluation of the esophageal diverticulum. The diverticu-

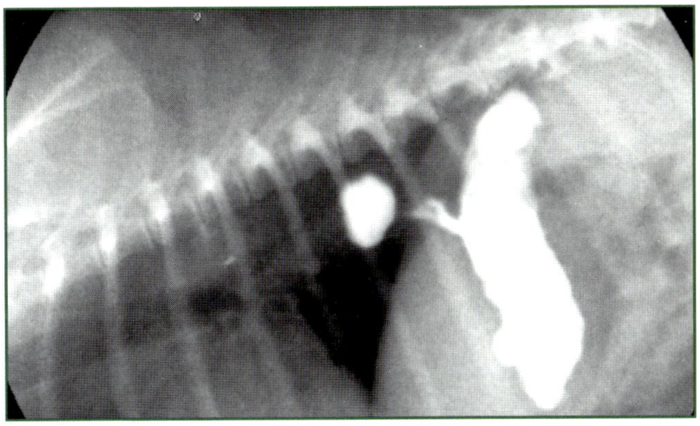

Figure 4.9 This esophagram shows retention of barium in a large esophageal diverticulum in the distal esophagus of a dog.

lum was resected, and the mucosal rent was closed. The dog made a complete recovery.

Comment

A pulsion diverticulum results secondary to mucosal disruption or weakening of the esophageal wall. Formation of epiphrenic diverticula and the relationship of esophageal foreign bodies has been described as an etiologic sequence in the dog.

Case 5

SIGNALMENT: 12-year-old male castrated Maltese dog

HISTORY: The dog was presented for a 6-week history of progressive regurgitation of undigested food immediately after eating. Changing the diet to a semiliquid consistency produced temporary relief. There was no improvement following cimetidine, antiemetic, and corticosteroid therapy. The owner had noted weight loss.

P.E.: The dog was thin but alert and active. Its temperature, pulse, and respiration rate were normal. The remainder of the physical examination was unremarkable.

ENDOSCOPIC FINDINGS: A 4 × 6-cm mass was visualized protruding into the lumen just cranial to the lower esophageal sphincter (*Figure 4.10*). The mucosal surface appeared normal.

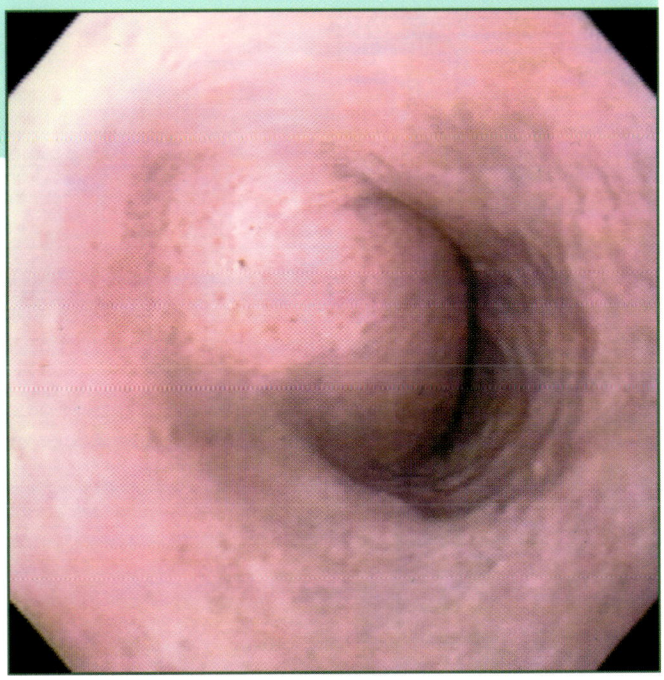

Figure 4.10 Endoscopic view of the distal esophagus showing a large submucosal mass protruding into the esophageal lumen just cranial to the lower esophageal sphincter.

Initial Assessment

Chronic regurgitation of food suggests esophageal disease. Expulsion of undigested food suggests an esophageal motility or obstructive disorder. The differential diagnosis includes megaesophagus, esophagitis, neoplasia, foreign body, esophageal stricture, or inflammatory esophageal disease. A barium contrast study would differentiate a megaesophagus from obstructive esophageal conditions. Endoscopy of the esophagus would be warranted to characterize obstructive lesions.

Presumptive Diagnosis

Esophageal disorder, possibly obstructive lesion or motility abnormality.

Diagnostic Plan

A CBC was normal, and the biochemical profile identified an elevated serum alkaline phosphatase value. This abnormality was attributed to previous corticosteroid therapy. Survey radiographs showed a dilated, gas-filled distal thoracic esophagus. Fluoroscopic examination of the esophagus was performed using a barium-sulfate suspension. Cranial to the lower esophageal sphincter was a transmural deviation of the esophageal lumen due to a focal, circumferential mass. A thin stream of barium was able to pass around the mass and enter the stomach. The esophagram was repeated using a food-barium mixture that showed obstruction of flow beyond the lesion.

Endoscopy identified a 4 × 6-cm mass protruding into the lumen at the level of the lower esophageal sphincter. The mucosal surface was normal and, when grasped with a biopsy forceps, the mucosa would slide over the surface of a submucosal mass. The mass was also evident from the gastric side of the lower esophageal sphincter. Two additional small (1-cm) submucosal masses were also identified in the fundic region of the stomach.

Outcome

The esophageal mass and the two gastric masses were removed during exploratory abdominal surgery. The masses were circumscribed and submucosal in location, thus, easily removed. Histopathology revealed that all of the resected masses were leiomyomas. The dog made an uneventful recovery, and all of its gastrointestinal signs resolved.

Comment

Esophageal leiomyomas occur most often at the level of the lower esophageal sphincter and, if large, can cause esophageal obstruction. Gastric leiomyomas also occur in the stomach but rarely cause clinical signs.

Case 6

SIGNALMENT: 4-month-old female Chinese shar-pei dog

HISTORY: This dog was presented for evaluation of acute episodes of regurgitation. The most recent episode had consisted of six bouts of regurgitation of undigested food, water, saliva, and mucus over a 24-hour period. The owner reported three similar episodes in the previous 2 months.

P.E.: The dog was lethargic and approximately 5% dehydrated. There was discomfort on palpation of the cranial abdomen.

ENDOSCOPIC FINDINGS: A view of the lower esophageal sphincter showed distal esophagitis with an open sphincter (*Figure 4.11*). Another view showed the lower esophageal sphincter from the stomach when distended with air (*Figure 4.12*). In *Figure 4.12*, the lower esophageal sphincter and cardia of the stomach are cranially displaced through an enlarged esophageal hiatus in the diaphragm. Imprints of the esophageal hiatus can be seen on the stomach wall.

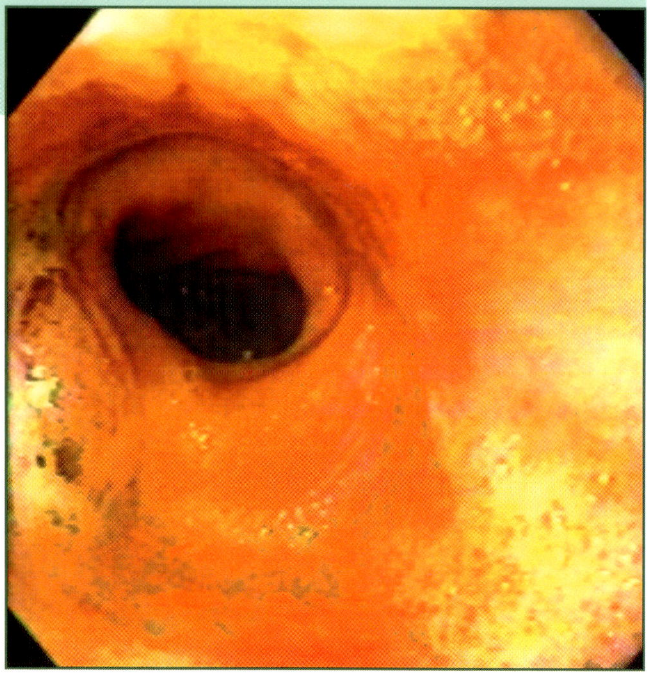

Figure 4.11 An endoscopic view showing the distal esophagus of a dog with esophagitis and an open lower esophageal sphincter.

Initial Assessment

The clinical presentation of acute regurgitation in a young dog suggests several esophageal disorders. Differentials for young dogs having esophageal disease include megaesophagus, foreign bodies, vascular ring anomalies, gastroesophageal intussusception, and hiatal hernia. The Chinese shar-pei breed has a higher incidence than other breeds of both megaesophagus and hiatal hernia. A foreign body is a less likely diagnosis because of the intermittent signs. Imaging studies, including plain thoracic radiographs and an esophagram, are indicated to evaluate the esophagus and lower esophageal sphincter. Endoscopy may be required to confirm the esophageal disorder.

Presumptive Diagnosis

Congenital megaesophagus, hiatal hernia, or gastroesophageal intussusception.

Diagnostic Plan

The dog was treated with intravenous fluids to correct dehydration. The results of a CBC, serum biochemical pro-

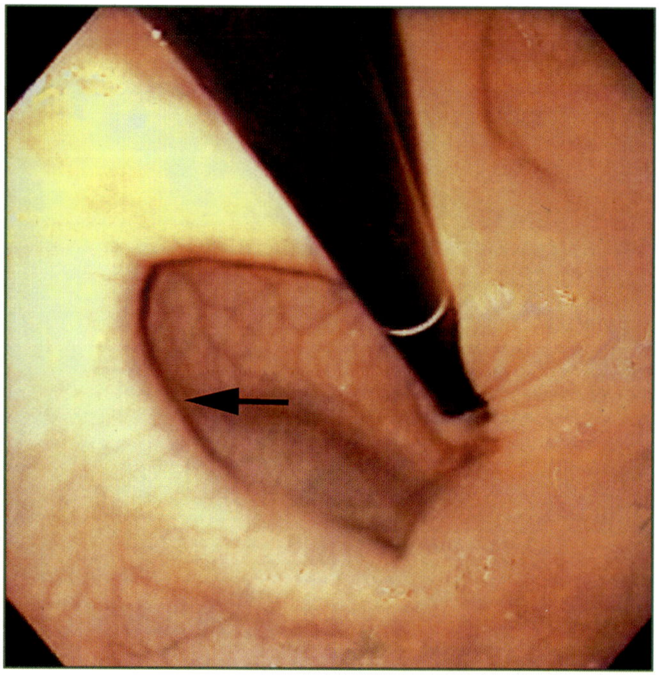

Figure 4.12 An endoscopic view of the lower esophageal sphincter viewed from the stomach. The lower esophageal sphincter and stomach are cranially displaced through an enlarged esophageal hiatus in the diaphragm. Imprints of the esophageal hiatus can be seen on the stomach wall (arrow).

file, and urinalysis were within normal limits. Survey thoracic radiographs showed a soft-tissue density in the caudal mediastinum. A liquid barium contrast esophagram demonstrated a dilated esophagus, with the lower esophageal sphincter and cardiac region of the stomach located within the caudal thorax (***Figure 4.13***).

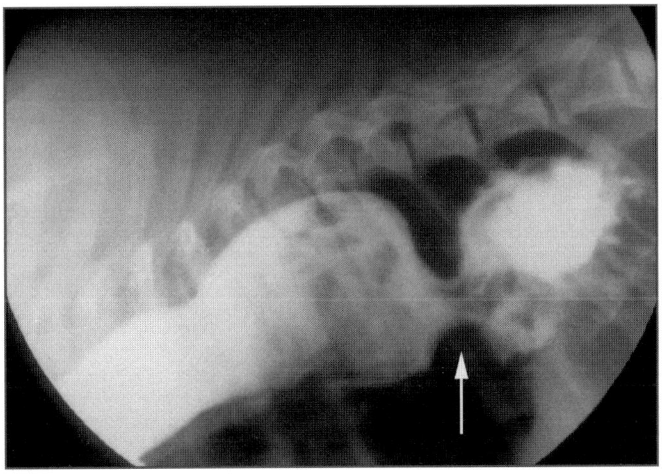

Figure 4.13 A barium esophagram showing a dilated esophagus with the lower esophageal sphincter (arrow) and fundic portion of the stomach herniated into the thorax.

Endoscopy identified distal esophagitis and an open lower esophageal sphincter. The endoscope was then advanced into the stomach; and, with the lumen distended, the tip of the scope was retroflexed to view the cardiac region and lower esophageal sphincter. Imprint of an abnormally large esophageal hiatus of the diaphragm can be seen in *Figure 4.13*, with the cardia and lower esophageal sphincter protruding through the defect and entering the thorax. A clinical diagnosis of a sliding hiatal hernia with secondary reflux esophagitis was made.

Outcome

During exploratory surgery, the stomach was returned to its normal position and a gastropexy was performed. The large esophageal hiatus of the diaphragm was then closed to a normal size. The dog recovered, and the problem of regurgitation resolved.

Comment

Sliding hiatal hernias are reported most often in the Chinese shar-pei, brachycephalic dogs, and cats. Clinical signs are most often due to incompetence of the lower esophageal sphincter with gastroesophageal reflux.

Case 7

SIGNALMENT: 5-year-old castrated male domestic shorthair cat

HISTORY: This cat was presented for chronic vomiting of 2 years' duration since it was obtained from a humane shelter. Its owner described almost daily vomiting of gastric fluid, mucus, and, occasionally, food. The vomiting was not related to eating; the cat was eating well and the owner reported that it was healthy in all other respects. Results of recent CBC, biochemical profile, fecal flotation, T_4, FIV, and FeLV tests were normal. Previous therapies for the vomiting included several hypoallergenic diets, febendazole, metronidazole, and prednisone—all without improvement.

P.E.: The physical examination was normal.

ENDOSCOPIC FINDINGS: An endoscopic view of the gastric body showed the mucosa was irregular and characterized by many prominent lymphoid follicles (*Figure 4.14*).

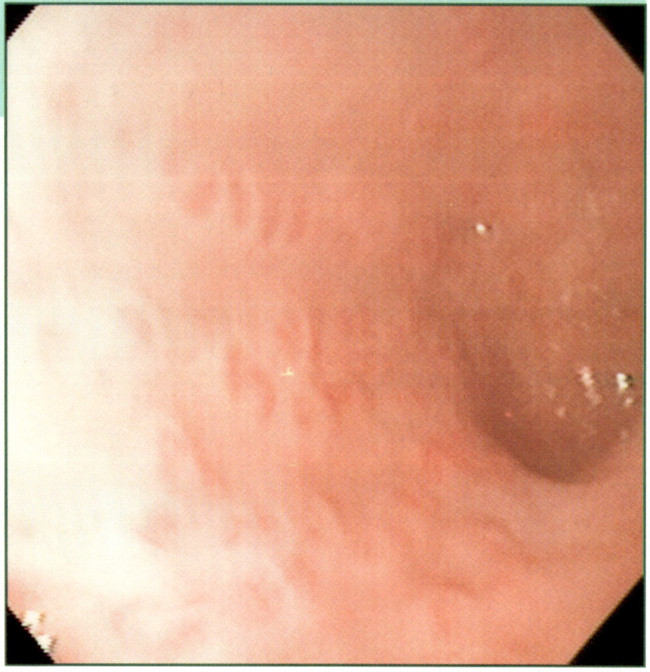

Figure 4.14 The endoscopic view of the body of the stomach in a cat showing an irregular mucosal surface due to prominent lymphoid follicles.

Initial Assessment

The main causes of chronic vomiting in cats include nongastrointestinal etiologies as well as gastrointestinal disorders. Major metabolic conditions were excluded based on previous laboratory testing. Dietary causes and parasites are less likely causes because of previous therapies. Likely etiologies include infectious or chronic inflammatory gastrointestinal disease. Vomiting is a common clinical sign of feline inflammatory bowel disease, which could be the cause in this case. Neoplasia or foreign bodies are less likely etiologies because of the chronic history. Further diagnostics are required to evaluate the gastrointestinal system; these include imaging techniques and endoscopy.

Presumptive Diagnosis

Primary gastrointestinal disease.

Diagnostic Plan

Routine abdominal radiographs were taken and were within normal limits. Abdominal ultrasound was performed to evaluate the gastrointestinal system, and the result was also considered normal. The next diagnostic step was endoscopy to evaluate both the stomach and proximal small intestine. Diffusely throughout the stomach were prominent lymphoid follicles giving the gastric mucosal surface a "cobblestone" appearance. Multiple specimens for biopsy, brush cytology, and urea culture for *Helicobacter* spp were collected. The small intestine appeared endoscopically normal, and biopsy samples were obtained. Histopathology confirmed lymphocytic follicular gastritis with *Helicobacter*-like organisms. Brush cytology confirmed the presence of multiple spiral bacteria (*Figure 4.15*), and the urea culture tube was positive for urease-forming bacteria. Histopathology of the intestine was normal.

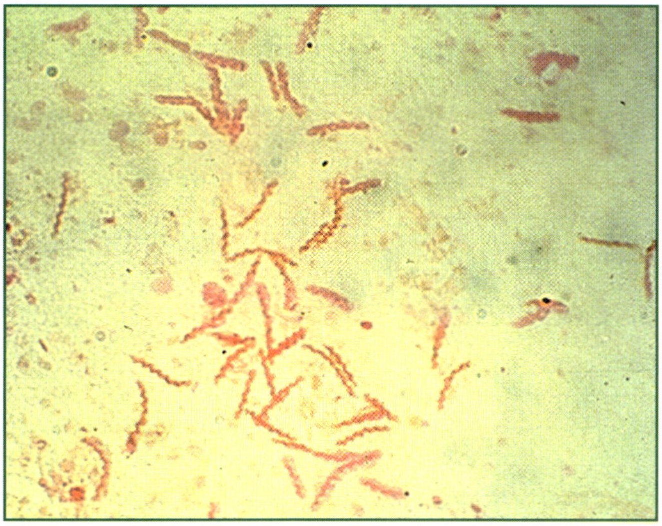

Figure 4.15 High-power oil immersion brush cytology of the gastric mucosa showing many spiral *Helicobacter* sp-like organisms (Gram's stain; ×100).

Outcome

With the clinical diagnosis of *Helicobacter*-sp gastritis, the cat was placed on a 2-week course of omeprazole, metronidazole, and amoxicillin. One week following therapy, the vomiting had resolved. Repeat gastroscopy performed 1 month after the therapy failed to demonstrate evidence of *Helicobacter* spp or gastritis.

Comment

Helicobacter-like organisms are common in the stomachs of dogs and cats, but the clinical significance of these organisms is still unclear. Regardless, evidence of gastritis and the presence of *Helicobacter*-like organisms should warrant trial therapy.

Case 8

SIGNALMENT: 6-year-old spayed female border terrier

HISTORY: This terrier was presented for chronic vomiting of approximately 6 months' duration. The owner described the occurrence of almost daily vomiting, mostly of food but occasionally gastric fluid. Vomiting of liquids was not reported to be a problem. The vomiting was described to occur shortly following a meal to many hours (more than 10 to 12) later. The dog was healthy in all other respects. The appetite was good, and there was no weight loss. No improvement occurred following either dietary or antiemetic trials.

P.E.: The physical examination was normal.

ENDOSCOPIC FINDINGS: An endoscopic view of the gastric antrum showed a large mucosal fold obstructing the pyloric opening (*Figure 4.16*).

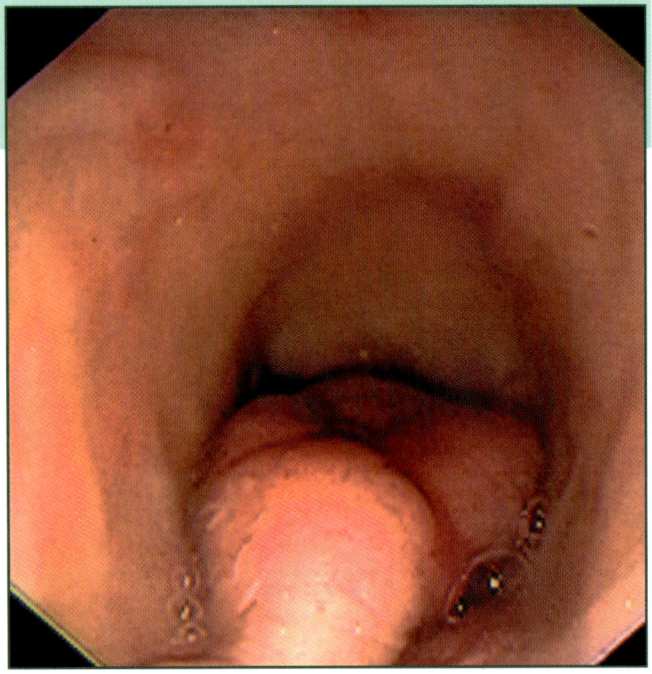

Figure 4.16 An endoscopic view showing the gastric antrum. There is a large mucosal fold obstructing the pyloric opening.

Initial Assessment

Chronic vomiting of food more than 10 hours after eating suggests a gastric outflow or motility disorder. In normal dogs, the stomach should be empty 8 to 10 hours after a meal. The differential diagnosis for vomiting in this case includes gastric foreign body, pyloric outflow obstruction, neoplasia, or gastric motility disorder. Malignant neoplasia would be less common; however, benign leiomyomas or polyps could cause delayed emptying. Hypertrophic pyloric gastropathy is a possible cause of gastric retention. Motility disorders can be either idiopathic or secondary to gastric disease. Systemic or metabolic disease is a less likely cause because of the chronic clinical signs.

Presumptive Diagnosis

Gastric outflow obstruction or gastric motility disorder.

Diagnostic Plan

Routine abdominal radiographs, a CBC, a biochemical profile, urinalysis, and fecal flotation were normal. To rule out morphologic gastric lesions, a gastrointestinal barium contrast study was performed. A large filling defect was found in the antrum of the stomach just proximal to the pylorus. Liquid barium was able to pass around the filling defect, however, and enter the intestine.

Endoscopy identified a large mucosal mass proximal to the pyloric opening. The endoscope passed around the mass and through the pylorus. The pyloric canal and proximal intestine were considered normal. Biopsy samples taken from the mass returned as normal gastric mucosa. Surgery identified the large mucosal fold in the antrum, which was resected; and a Y-U pyloroplasty was performed to open the pyloric canal.

Outcome

Histopathology confirmed the diagnosis of mucosal hypertrophy. Following surgery, the chronic vomiting resolved.

Comment

A syndrome of hypertrophic pyloric gastropathy is associated with benign pyloric lesions, resulting in gastric outlet obstruction. This syndrome is most often associated with hypertrophic mucosal folds or "polyps" that obstruct the pyloric lumen. The condition is reported to occur most commonly in small-breed dogs and is often responsive to surgical techniques for correction of the outflow obstruction.

Case 9

SIGNALMENT: 5-year-old castrated male collie-mix dog
HISTORY: This dog was presented for chronic intermittent vomiting of 3 months' duration. The vomitus consisted of gastric fluid and, sometimes, bile. The dog was vomiting approximately two to three times a week. Vomiting was not associated with eating. The appetite was good, and the dog was healthy in all other respects. Multiple therapies, including antibiotics, dietary trials, antiemetics, and corticosteroids, had failed to resolve the problem.
P.E.: The physical examination was normal.
ENDOSCOPIC FINDINGS: A view of the gastric body showed a parasite embedded in the gastric mucosa (*Figure 4.17*).

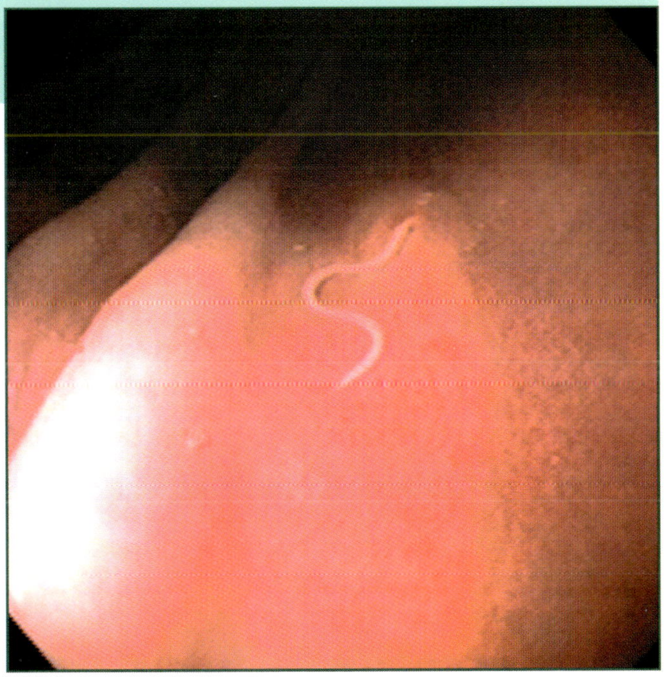

Figure 4.17 An endoscopic view of the body of the canine stomach showing a *Physaloptera* sp embedded in the mucosa.

Initial Assessment

Chronic intermittent vomiting is a common clinical complaint. After systemic or metabolic disease has been ruled out, the differential diagnosis focuses on gastrointestinal problems. Dietary, inflammatory, infectious, and neoplastic diseases should be considered. Infectious causes include *Helicobacter* spp and gastrointestinal parasites, such as *Giardia* or *Physaloptera* spp or ascarids. A chronic gastric foreign body is also possible.

Presumptive Diagnosis

Gastric or intestinal disease, most likely gastritis.

Diagnostic Plan

A routine CBC, biochemical profile, urinalysis, and fecal flotation were performed. Mild peripheral eosinophilia was identified, which suggested possible dietary allergies or parasites. A heartworm test was negative. Further evaluation involved imaging studies, including routine abdominal radiographs and abdominal ultrasound, and both were within normal limits. Gastrointestinal endoscopy identified a *Physaloptera*-sp helminth attached to the mucosa in the greater curvature of the stomach. The parasite was endoscopically removed and identified. Results of a biopsy of the gastric mucosa returned as mild eosinophilic gastritis. The duodenum was normal.

Outcome

The dog was treated with the anthelmintic febendazole and, following therapy, the vomiting resolved.

Comment

Physaloptera sp is a gastric parasite that causes chronic vomiting but is difficult to diagnose. Fecal flotation with detection of ova is frequently unrewarding, while endoscopy with direct visualization of the helminths confirms the diagnosis. Therapy using anthelmintics, such as febendazole or pyrantel pamoate, eliminates the parasite.

Case 10

SIGNALMENT: 11-year-old castrated male chow chow dog

HISTORY: The dog was presented for anorexia, weight loss, and chronic vomiting of 1 month's duration. The owner described the vomitus as often containing flecks of either fresh or digested blood. Episodes of vomiting had increased to several times a day. The dog's appetite was poor, and the dog was unresponsive to antacid therapy using famotidine. Occasionally, the stool was dark in color. There was no concurrent drug therapy, and no other systemic signs were noted.

P.E.: The dog was weak and thin. Mucous membranes were pale in color. Abdominal palpation was unremarkable.

ENDOSCOPIC FINDINGS: An endoscopic view of the gastric angle showed a thickened wall with deep ulcers (*Figure 4.18*).

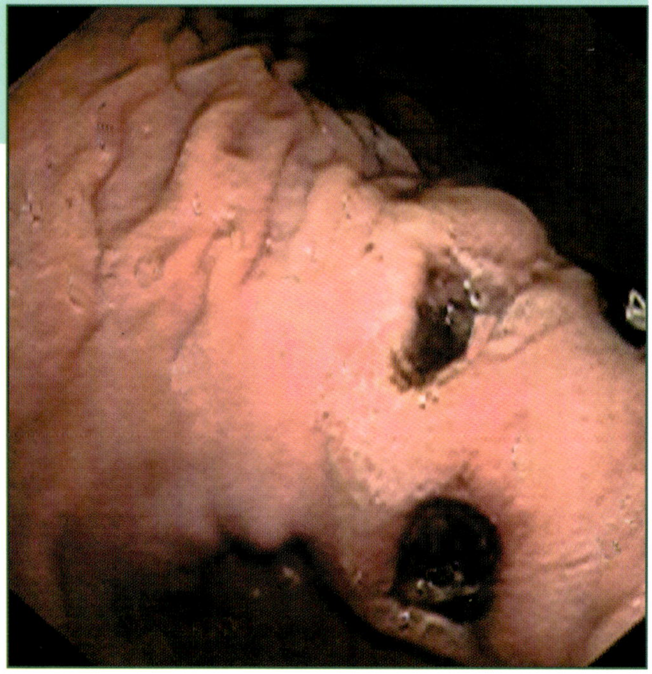

Figure 4.18 An endoscopic view showing the area of the gastric angle of the stomach. The gastric wall is rigid and thickened and has two deep mucosal ulcers.

Initial Assessment

The history of vomiting blood combined with passing dark stools suggests gastric ulceration. The cause of ulceration in this case could be associated with neoplasia; a foreign body; or a metabolic disorder, such as hypoadrenocorticism, renal failure, or liver disease. A gastrinoma, or gastrin-secreting tumor, can result in increased gastric acid production and subsequent gastric ulceration. Drugs, such as nonsteroidal anti-inflammatory agents, cause gastric ulcers; however, there is no history of drug therapy in this case. Chronic gastritis or *Helicobacter* spp are also possible causes of ulceration. Concurrent signs of anorexia with weight loss suggest serious disease, such as neoplasia.

Presumptive Diagnosis

Gastric ulceration, possibly neoplasia.

Diagnostic Plan

A minimum database, including CBC, biochemical profile, and urinalysis, was obtained. Abnormalities found were a mild microcytic anemia, hypoproteinemia, and hypokalemia. The anemia and hypoproteinemia are most likely associated with gastrointestinal blood loss. A fecal examination was negative for parasites but positive for occult blood, documenting gastrointestinal bleeding. Thoracic radiographs were negative for metastasis, and abdominal radiographs were unremarkable. Abdominal ultrasound showed a thickened gastric wall and enlarged gastric lymph nodes.

Endoscopy of the stomach identified a thickened gastric angle and lesser curvature with two areas of mucosal ulceration. The thickened region of the stomach was rigid and nondistensible. Multiple biopsy specimens were taken at the margin of the ulcer. Attempts were made to repeat biopsy sampling in the same site to obtain deeper submucosal tissue. Histopathology confirmed adenocarcinoma.

Outcome

Because of the extensive involvement of the gastric adenocarcinoma and the poor prognosis, the owner requested euthanasia.

Comments

Adenocarcinoma is the most common gastric tumor in the dog. Frequently, the tumor invades submucosally, sometimes with minimal mucosal disruption, thus requiring a deep submucosal biopsying technique to make the diagnosis.

Case 11

SIGNALMENT: 4-year-old female Yorkshire terrier dog

HISTORY: The dog presented with a 3-week history of watery, small-bowel diarrhea. Its appetite was good, although weight loss had been noted by the owner. Initial laboratory tests previously performed indicated significant hypoproteinemia. The dog was treated with metronidazole but did not respond to the therapy.

P.E.: The dog was alert and active. There was abdominal distention from suspected fluid. The remainder of the physical examination was unremarkable.

ENDOSCOPIC FINDINGS: An endoscopic view of the proximal duodenum showed prominent, white, villous tips in the intestine (*Figure 4.19*).

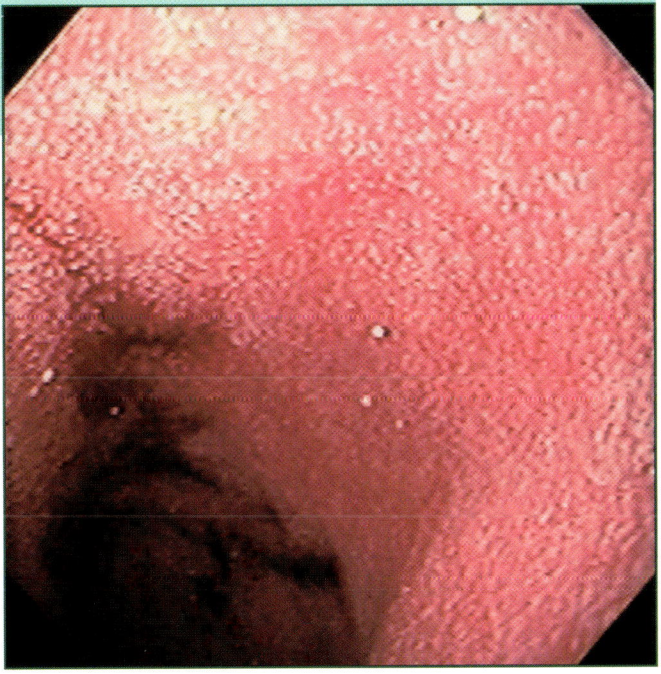

Figure 4.19 An endoscopic view showing the proximal duodenum of a dog. Note the prominent white villous tips of the intestinal mucosa, which are characteristic of lymphatic dilation.

Initial Assessment

Chronic small-bowel diarrhea and weight loss that occur with a good appetite suggest either a malabsorption or maldigestion disorder. The historical evidence of hypoproteinemia suggests a possible protein-losing enteropathy. Differential diagnosis for a protein-losing enteropathy includes inflammatory bowel disease, intestinal neoplasia, granulomatous enteritis, fungal disease, and lymphangiectasia. Yorkshire terriers are reported to be at increased risk for lymphangiectasia. The suspected abdominal fluid detected on physical examination is most likely the result of the hypoproteinemia. Causes for hypoproteinemia include starvation, liver disease, and losses through the gastrointestinal tract and kidney or from sequestration of protein in a body cavity.

Presumptive Diagnosis

Protein-losing enteropathy.

Diagnostic Plan

A minimum database was established, including a CBC, a biochemical profile, urinalysis, fecal flotation, and fecal cytology. Serum bile acid tests were performed to evaluate liver function. Abnormalities included a lymphopenia, nonregenerative anemia, and a marked panhypoproteinemia. Normal liver function and lack of renal protein loss supports the presumptive diagnosis of a protein-losing enteropathy. Thoracic radiographs were normal. Abdominal ultrasound confirmed marked abdominal effusion, thickened small bowel, and prominent mesenteric lymph nodes. Abdominocentesis was performed next, yielding a clear and colorless fluid that was determined to be a transudate. Fecal examinations were normal. Upper gastrointestinal endoscopy was performed to determine the cause of the gastrointestinal protein loss. The gastric mucosa appeared edematous. The surface of the duodenum had prominent villous tips with a whitish appearance suggestive of lymphatic dilation. Histopathology confirmed

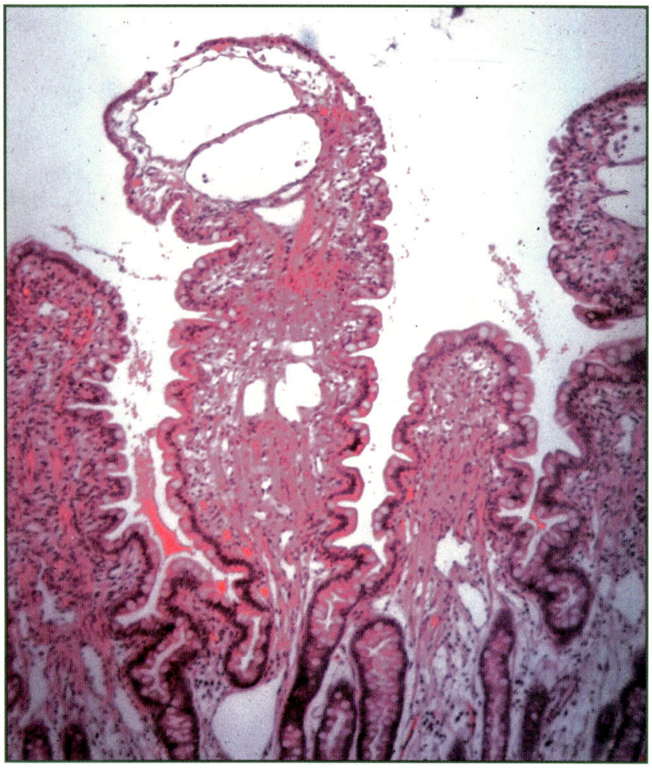

Figure 4.20 Histopathology of the duodenal mucosal biopsy showing dilated lymphatics characteristic of lymphangiectasia in the intestinal villi. (H&E stain; ×40)

lymphangiectasia with dilated lacteals and mild lymphocytic plasmacytic enteritis (***Figure 4.20***).

Outcome

The lymphangiectasia was treated with a low-fat diet that contained medium-chain triglycerides and anti-inflammatory doses of prednisolone. Rutin, a bioflavonoid reported to be of benefit for lymphedema, was included in the therapy. A 3-week course of the antibiotic tylosin was also prescribed for possible secondary bacterial overgrowth. The diarrhea resolved, and protein concentration slowly increased. The prednisolone was tapered over time, and the dog was maintained on a low-fat diet.

Comment

Lymphangiectasia can occur as either a primary disorder or secondary to obstructive lesions in the lymphatics. Lymphatic stasis results in loss of lymph into the intestine, with loss of fat (triglycerides), protein, and lymphocytes. Therapy includes reduction of dietary fat to decrease lymphatic flow to the intestine and, hence, a reduced lymphatic loss through the dilated lacteals. Anti-inflammatory drugs and rutin may be of benefit. The prognosis is guarded, especially when total protein concentrations drop below 3 mg/dl.

Case 12

SIGNALMENT: 12-year-old castrated male domestic shorthair cat

HISTORY: The cat was presented for chronic intermittent vomiting of approximately 3 months' duration. The owner described the signs as more pronounced during the few weeks before presentation. Appetite had decreased, there was evidence of weight loss, and the vomiting had increased in frequency. Previous therapies included dietary trials, febendazole for possible parasites, and several courses of antibiotics.

P.E.: Temperature, pulse, and respiratory rate were within the normal range. The cat was thin and had an unkempt haircoat. Its intestines felt thickened on abdominal palpation.

ENDOSCOPIC FINDINGS: An endoscopic view of the descending duodenum showed an irregular duodenal mucosa with a focal area of mucosal ulceration and hemorrhage (*Figure 4.21*).

Initial Assessment

With the cat's history of chronic vomiting, both gastrointestinal disorders and systemic or metabolic disease are possible. In older cats, hyperthyroidism and renal disease should always be investigated through laboratory testing. Because of the palpably thickened intestine and prominent mesenteric lymph nodes, intestinal disorders, such as inflammatory bowel disease or neoplasia (such as lymphoma), are possible. Gastric disorders, such as gastritis, *Helicobacter*-sp infection, neoplasia, or foreign bodies, can cause vomiting but are less likely diagnoses based on the current physical findings.

Presumptive Diagnosis

Intestinal disease.

Diagnostic Plan

A minimum database, including a CBC, a biochemical profile, and urinalysis, should be obtained. In cats, additional database tests should include FeLV, FIV, and T_4. The

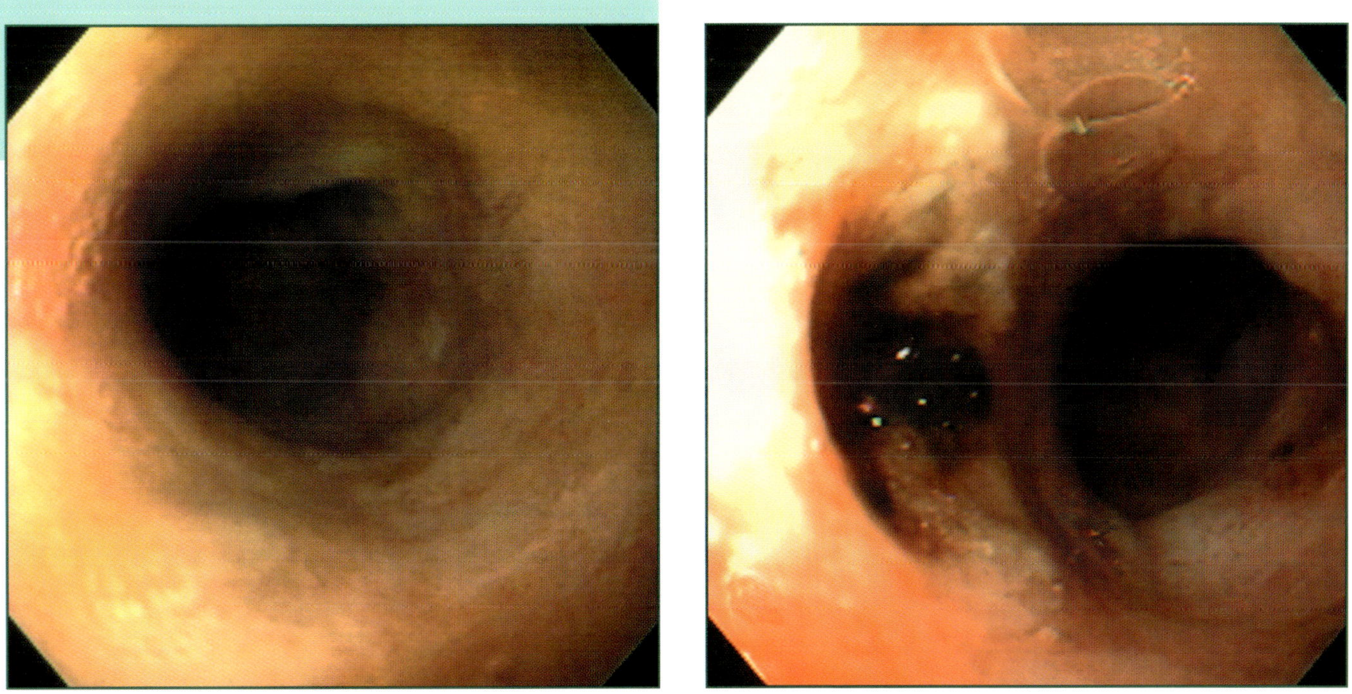

Figure 4.21 Left, The endoscopic view showing the proximal duodenum of a cat previously diagnosed to have inflammatory bowel disease. The mucosa is slightly irregular, and a mucosal ulcer can be seen at approximately the 9 o'clock location in the lumen. Right, The close-up view of the duodenal ulcer in a cat with inflammatory bowel disease.

CBC showed a mild inflammatory leukocytosis and a nonregenerative anemia. The remainder of the initial laboratory values were normal. Because of the high probability of intestinal disease, fecal flotation and fecal cytology were performed and were negative. Ultrasound evaluation of the gastrointestinal tract showed thickening of the small intestine and enlargement of mesenteric lymph nodes.

At this point in the workup, clinicians believed intestinal biopsy was indicated to determine the cause of the intestinal thickening. Endoscopy was performed to evaluate the stomach and upper small intestine. The stomach appeared normal; however, the duodenal mucosa was hyperemic and had an irregular luminal surface. There were also three distinct focal areas of ulceration approximately 3 mm in diameter. These areas appeared to have necrotic or hemorrhagic centers. Multiple biopsy specimens were taken from the mucosa and at the margins of the ulcers. Histopathology identified a marked lymphocytic plasmacytic infiltrate with villous atrophy. Biopsy of the ulcers produced necrotic material with many neutrophils and bacteria.

Outcome

A diagnosis of inflammatory bowel disease with secondary necrotic ulcers was made. Because the ulcers were thought to be secondary to a bacterial origin, the cat was treated with a 3-week course of amoxicillin and enrofloxacin. The inflammatory bowel disease was treated using dietary modification and anti-inflammatory therapy with prednisolone. The incidence of vomiting decreased, and the appetite improved.

Comment

Vomiting, rather than diarrhea, is frequently the primary clinical sign in feline small intestinal inflammatory disease. A definitive diagnosis requires an intestinal biopsy. The ulceration in focal necrotic areas that were observed in this case is an uncommon complication of inflammatory bowel disease.

Case 13

SIGNALMENT: 12-year-old spayed female Lhasa apso dog
HISTORY: The owner presented this dog after it vomited intermittently for 3 weeks. The vomitus consisted predominately of bilious fluid, the dog's appetite was poor, and the vomiting was not associated with eating. The dog was not receiving therapy.
P.E.: The physical examination was unremarkable.
ENDOSCOPIC FINDINGS: An endoscopic view of the proximal duodenum showed normal-appearing mucosa (*Figure 4.22*). However, the endoscopic view of the duodenum 17 cm beyond the pylorus showed narrowing of the lumen due to a white, fibrouslike lesion (*Figure 4.23*). The lumen narrowed to approximately 5 mm in diameter, which was too small to allow passing the endoscope beyond that point.

Initial Assessment

Bilious vomiting is often a sign of gastric hypomotility with reflux of bile back into the stomach. The gastric hypomotility is either secondary to gastric disease or occurs because of a primary idiopathic motility disorder (idiopathic bilious vomiting syndrome). Other causes of bilious vomiting could include inflammatory and obstructive disorders of the proximal intestine. Such conditions as *Giardia* or *Physaloptera* infection or inflammatory bowel disease are the most common intestinal disorders that can result in bilious vomiting. The poor appetite in this case may suggest a more significant gastrointestinal disorder than idiopathic bilious vomiting syndrome. Certain systemic or metabolic disease could also result in vomiting.

Presumptive Diagnosis

Idiopathic bilious vomiting.

Diagnostic Plan

A minimum database including a CBC, a biochemical profile, urinalysis, and fecal flotation was established and

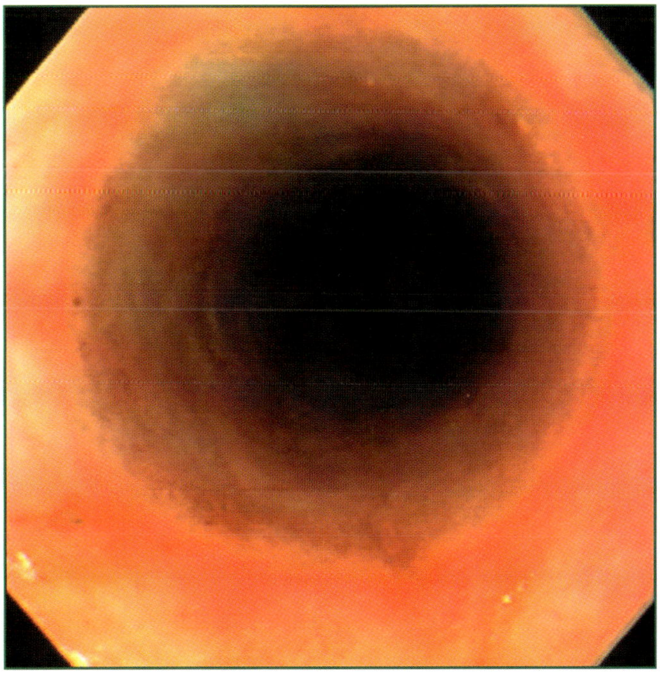

Figure 4.22 Endoscopic view of the proximal duodenum of a dog showing hyperemic mucosa.

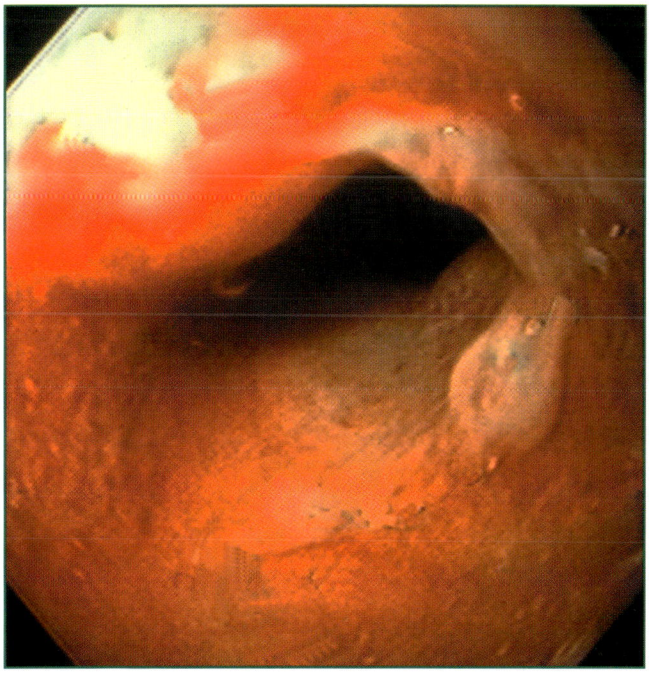

Figure 4.23 Endoscopic view of the duodenum 17 cm beyond the pylorus showing narrowing of the lumen due to a white, firm, fibrouslike lesion.

all values were normal. Routine abdominal radiographs were taken to rule out obvious gastrointestinal disorders, radiopaque foreign bodies, or other intra-abdominal abnormalities. Based on the negative initial workup, upper gastrointestinal endoscopy was performed as the next diagnostic test. The stomach and the proximal duodenum appeared endoscopically normal. Approximately 17 cm caudal to the pylorus was a narrowing of the luminal diameter to approximately 5 mm, caused by a firm, white, fibrous lesion. The endoscope could not be passed beyond this lesion. Multiple biopsy specimens were taken at the margin of the lesion as well as at the normal-looking proximal duodenum and stomach. Histopathology of the duodenal lesion confirmed intestinal adenocarcinoma.

Outcome

Thoracic radiographs were taken to evaluate for metastasis and were negative. Exploratory surgery was performed, and the lesion was identified. A wide surgical resection of the adenocarcinoma lesion was done (***Figure 4.24***). There was no gross evidence of metastasis, and histopathology of the regional lymph nodes was negative for metastasis. The dog made an uneventful recovery and was euthanized 2 years later for causes unrelated to this condition.

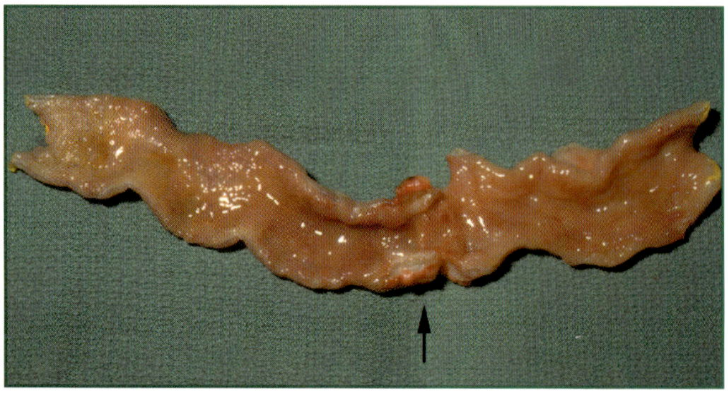

Figure 4.24 The surgically resected duodenal adenocarcinoma (arrow) was diagnosed endoscopically.

Comment

Adenocarcinoma of the small intestine is uncommon in dogs. The lesions tend to occur as annular constrictions of the intestinal wall, producing signs associated with a partial obstruction. Vomiting and weight loss are frequent presenting clinical complaints.

Case 14

SIGNALMENT: 12-year-old spayed female Persian cat

HISTORY: The owner presented the cat for chronic diarrhea of 2 years' duration. The diarrhea had previously been diagnosed as probable inflammatory bowel disease but had never been confirmed by biopsy. The cat was managed using various dietary trials and intermittent courses of prednisolone. During the 2 months prior to presentation, however, significant lethargy, diarrhea, and weight loss developed. The cat's appetite was poor, and the diarrhea was unresponsive to a change in diet. The cat was negative for feline leukemia virus and feline immunodeficiency virus, and thyroid function was normal.

P.E.: Temperature, pulse, and respiratory rate were normal. The cat appeared lethargic, had pale membranes, and was very thin. Abdominal palpation identified a fluid-filled small intestine.

ENDOSCOPIC FINDINGS: An endoscopic view of the proximal small intestine showed the mucosa had a prominent villous surface (*Figure 4.25*).

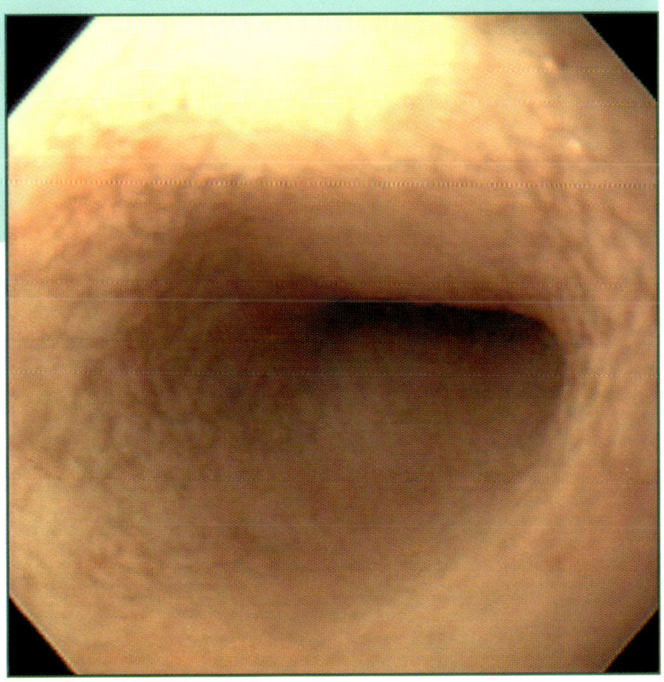

Figure 4.25 An endoscopic view of the proximal small intestine in a cat. The mucosa has a prominent villous surface.

Initial Assessment

The cat had previously been diagnosed clinically as having inflammatory bowel disease and was controlled using dietary manipulation. The diarrhea and weight loss before presentation first suggested a relapse in the inflammatory bowel disease. Relapses are common and often require aggressive therapy. *There is evidence that inflammatory bowel disease can sometimes progress to intestinal lymphoma.* The probability of gastrointestinal lymphoma is also likely because of the recent clinical deterioration. Other gastrointestinal conditions, such as bacterial overgrowth, exocrine pancreatic insufficiency, intestinal adenocarcinoma, or other unrelated systemic or metabolic disease, should also be considered.

Presumptive Diagnosis

Relapse of inflammatory bowel disease.

Diagnostic Plan

A minimum database, including a CBC, a biochemical profile, and urinalysis was established and identified a mild nonregenerative anemia. Fecal flotation, fecal cytology, and a *Cryptosporidium* sp-sensitive, fecal ELISA were negative. Because significant systemic and metabolic disease had been ruled out by initial testing, further investigation of the gastrointestinal tract was indicated. Additional diagnostics included an abdominal ultrasound as well as serum cobalamin, folate, and feline trypsin-like immunoreactivity (fTLI) tests. A barium contrast study was not performed in this case.

Abdominal ultrasound showed diffuse thickening of the intestinal wall and mild mesenteric lymphadenopathy. Cobalamin concentrations were below the normal reference range. Low cobalamin levels frequently occur secondary to gastrointestinal, liver, or pancreatic disease. At this point in

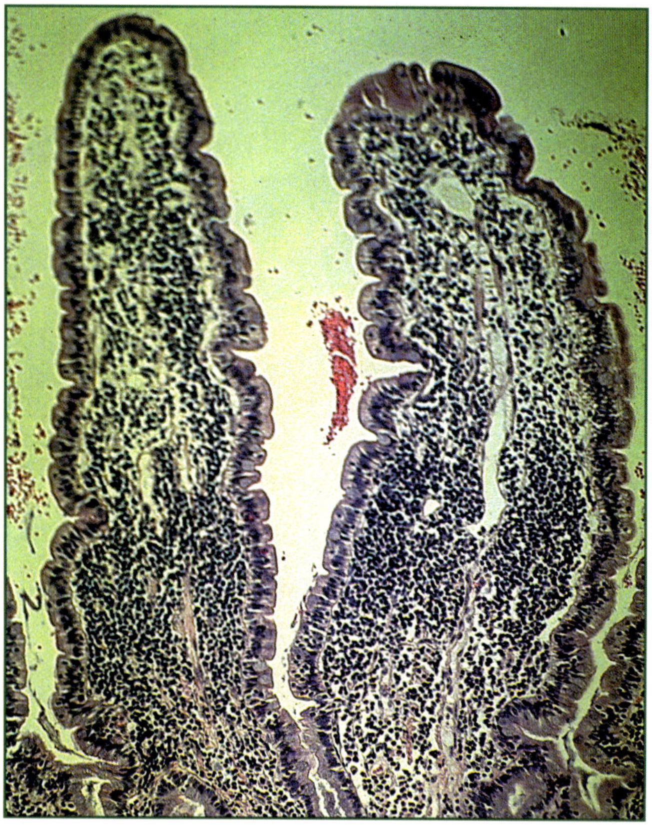

Figure 4.26 Histopathology of the endoscopic biopsy showing diffuse lymphocytic lymphoma in the intestinal villi. (H&E stain; ×40)

the workup, intestinal biopsy was indicated to confirm the type of intestinal disease in this cat. Endoscopy was performed, and the proximal small intestine appeared to be of normal color with no significant mucosal surface irregularities. The intestinal villi were prominent and appeared to be swollen. Multiple intestinal biopsy specimens were obtained. Histopathology confirmed diffuse intestinal lymphocytic lymphoma (***Figure 4.26***).

Outcome

The cat was treated with prednisolone, chlorambucil, and cobalamin replacement. It remained in remission on therapy for 10 months, after which the signs reoccurred. The owner declined further therapy, and the cat was euthanized.

Comment

It is relatively common for the endoscopic appearance of the intestine in either inflammatory bowel disease or intestinal lymphocytic lymphoma to show minimal to no gross mucosal changes. There is also evidence that inflammatory disease can progress to gastrointestinal lymphoma. In some cases, it is difficult to differentiate severe inflammatory bowel disease from lymphoma histologically and full-thickness surgical biopsy may be indicated.

Case 15

SIGNALMENT: 1-year-old castrated male mixed-breed dog.

HISTORY: This dog was presented for 3 months' duration of chronic diarrhea that was characterized by increased urgency, frequency, and tenesmus. The stool frequently contained fresh blood and, occasionally, mucus. At the onset of diarrhea, the dog was diagnosed as having whipworms and was treated with febendazole. The clinical signs continued, however. Other trial therapies included a high-fiber diet, metronidazole, prednisone, and tylosin.

P.E.: The dog was alert and active. The temperature, pulse, and respiratory rate were normal. There was evidence of abdominal discomfort on palpation. A rectal examination was negative, but the stool was soft and contained small flecks of blood.

ENDOSCOPIC FINDINGS: The endoscopic view in the proximal ascending colon showed a tissue mass projecting into the lumen (*Figure 4.27*).

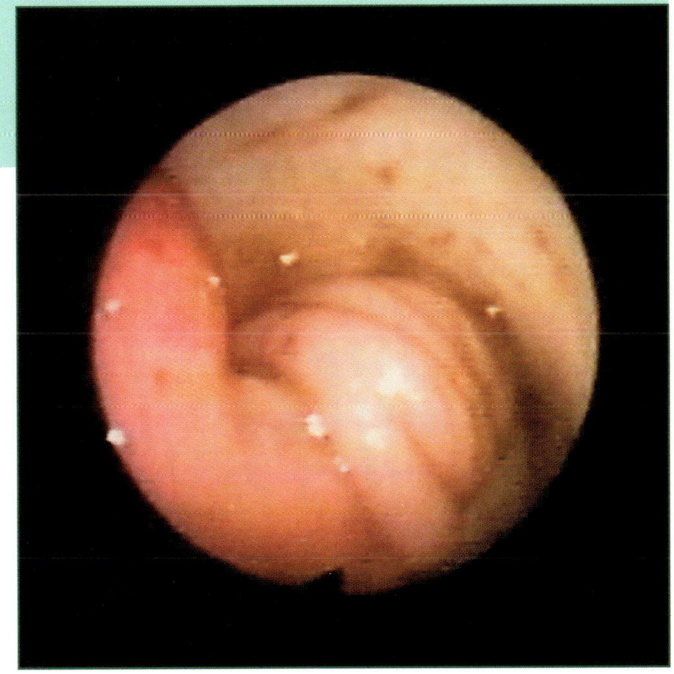

Figure 4.27 Endoscopic view in the proximal ascending colon showing a tissue mass projecting into the lumen. The mucosal surface of the mass appears normal.

Initial Assessment

This dog's clinical signs are characteristic of large-bowel diarrhea. The presence of hematochezia suggests mucosal ulceration. Intestinal parasites should be considered but are unlikely because of the recent anthelmintic therapy. Other causes of colonic disease include various types of colitis, polyps, tumors, or strictures. The abdominal discomfort detected on physical examination may be associated with the suspected colonic disease or other intra-abdominal disorders.

Presumptive Diagnosis

Chronic colitis.

Diagnostic Plan

A minimum database was established to rule out involvement of systemic disease and was normal. Fecal flotation was performed and was negative for parasites. Cytologic examination of the feces using Diff-Quik stain showed a slight increase in neutrophil numbers, suggesting inflammation or an infectious etiology. Abdominal radiographs were taken because of the abdominal discomfort detected and showed gas distention of the ascending colon, which contained fecal material. With the chronic large-bowel signs exhibited by this patient, colonoscopy was deemed relevant. No obvious abnormalities were identified on examination of the descending and transverse portions of the colon. In the ascending colon, there was a large polypoid mass protruding into the lumen at the level of the cecum. The ileocolic valve was identified, located adjacent to the tissue mass. Biopsy of the mass was done, and histopathology confirmed normal mucosa. The diagnosis was a cecal inversion.

Outcome

Surgery confirmed the presence of a cecal inversion, and it was removed. The dog made an uneventful recovery, and its chronic diarrhea resolved.

Comment

Cecal inversion (or cecocolic invagination) is uncommon but, when it occurs, is most frequently associated with the presence of whipworms. The diagnosis can be made through barium contrast studies, by ultrasound showing a mass in the region of the cecum, or by visualizing the inversion using flexible fiberoptic endoscopy.

Case 16

SIGNALMENT: 10-year-old castrated male golden retriever dog

HISTORY: This dog presented with a 3-week history of blood-streaked stools. The blood was fresh and the owner reported there were no signs of tenesmus, urgency, or increased frequency of stool passage. The dog was described as in excellent health otherwise.

P.E.: The dog was alert and active. A complete physical examination was unremarkable. Rectal examination identified a small amount of blood associated with the feces. The anal glands were not distended.

ENDOSCOPIC FINDINGS: An endoscopic view from the colon was obtained with the endoscope retroflexed caudally to view the rectum (*Figure 4.28*). Two polypoid lesions were identified protruding into the rectal lumen.

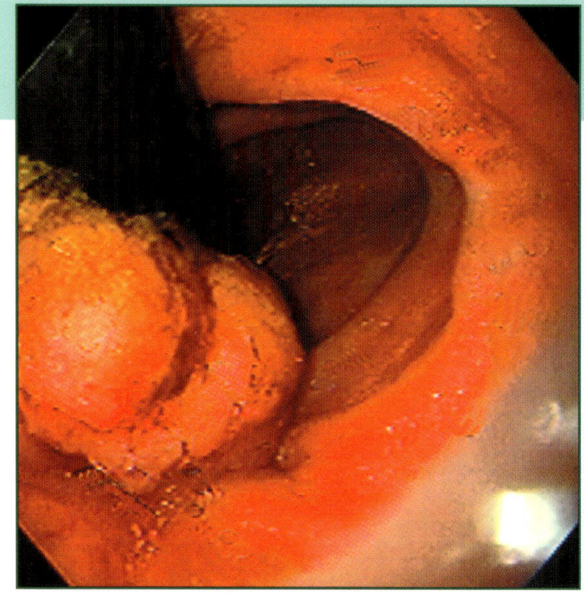

Figure 4.28 Endoscopic view from the colon of a dog with the endoscopic tip retroflexed into the J position viewing distally to the rectum. Two polypoid lesions are visible protruding into the rectal lumen.

Initial Assessment

The dog was presented for hematochezia. Rectal bleeding could be associated with a coagulation disorder but is unlikely because there were no other areas of bleeding noted. Other causes of bleeding include anal sac disease, colitis, polyps, tumors, or ulcers. Anal sac disease is unlikely because of the normal rectal examination. Colitis is often associated with other signs, including tenesmus, frequency, and urgency. Fecal mucus is also often present with colitis. Parasites are possible but unlikely in older dogs. In the older dog, polyps or tumors are possible etiologies.

Presumptive Diagnosis

Colonic or rectal bleeding; possibly colitis, tumors, or polyps.

Diagnostic Plan

A CBC, biochemical profile, and urinalysis were completed, and all results were within normal limits. Fecal flotation and fecal cytology were also normal. Abdominal radiographs were taken and were considered to be normal. A careful evaluation was made for enlargement of sublumbar lymph nodes that could result from metastasis of colonic or rectal neoplasia. Ultrasound evaluation of the gastrointestinal tract is helpful in identifying infiltrative inflammatory or neoplastic intestinal lesions but was not performed in this case.

The dog was prepared for colonoscopy using enemas and a colonic lavage solution. To perform the procedure, the endoscope was advanced through the rectum and the lumen insufflated with air. The entire colon was felt to be normal. While withdrawing the endoscope, mucosal biopsy specimens were obtained. In the distal descending colon, the endoscopic tip was retroflexed caudally 190° to view the rectum. Two polypoid lesions were observed protruding into the lumen. Mucosal biopsies of the masses were performed, and findings were consistent with inflammatory polyps.

Outcome

A large, bi-lobed inflammatory polyp was surgically removed by prolapsing rectal mucosa to the level of the polyps. Histology of the mass confirmed the diagnosis of an inflammatory polyp.

Comment

Intestinal polyps in dogs most frequently occur in the rectal region of the gastrointestinal tract. Many can be palpated during rectal examination. Hematochezia is the most frequent clinical sign. Colorectal polyps are best viewed endoscopically by retroflexing the endoscope caudally while in the distal descending colon.

Case 17

SIGNALMENT: 6-year-old intact female Welsh terrier

HISTORY: This dog was presented after 3 weeks of chronic diarrhea. The diarrhea was described as frequent episodes of small mucoid stools. Tenesmus was also present. There was no weight loss, and the appetite was good. The owner stated that the dog had had no previous medical problems.

P.E.: The dog was alert and active. The temperature, pulse, and heart rate were normal. Abdominal palpation was unremarkable. The rectal examination was normal, and the stool was of a mucoid consistency.

ENDOSCOPIC FINDINGS: In an endoscopic view of the descending colon, the mucosal surface was granular in appearance and there was lack of normal submucosal blood vessels (*Figure 4.29*).

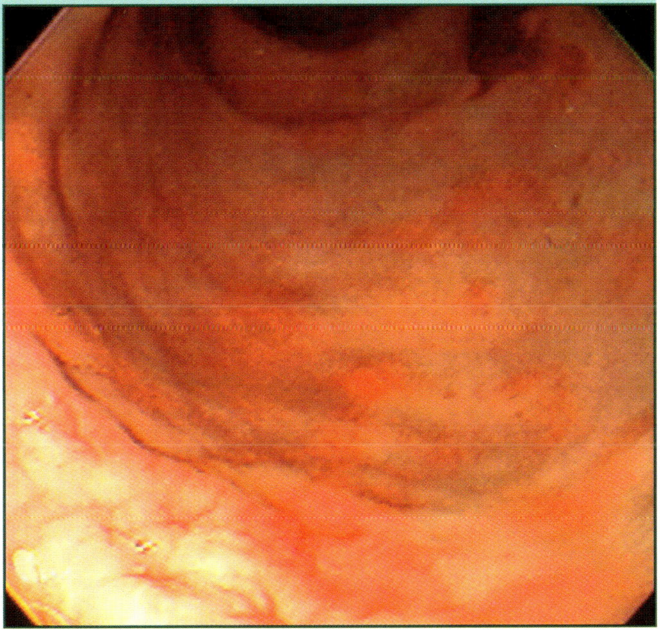

Figure 4.29 Endoscopic view of the descending colon of a dog. The mucosal surface is granular in appearance and shows a lack of normal submucosal blood vessels, suggesting mucosal inflammatory infiltrates.

Initial Assessment

The dog presented for signs of chronic, large-bowel diarrhea. Lack of weight loss or other systemic signs suggests primary colonic disease. Conditions causing large-bowel diarrhea include parasites, chronic colitis, granulomatous colitis, neoplasia, polyps, and strictures. Parasites, such as whipworms, should always be considered but are a less likely finding than other causes in a 6-year-old dog. Chronic colitis is likely, but requires biopsy to confirm the presence and type of inflammatory infiltrates. Lymphocytic-plasmacytic and eosinophilic infiltrates are the most common types associated with colitis in the dog. Fungal disease is unlikely because of the environmental geographical location. Neoplasia, granulomatous colitis, and colonic strictures are uncommon.

Presumptive Diagnosis

Colonic disease, possibly chronic colitis.

Diagnostic Plan

A minimum database was determined to eliminate possible metabolic or systemic disease as the cause of the large-bowel diarrhea. The CBC identified peripheral eosinophilia that suggested either gastrointestinal parasites or allergic colitis. A fecal flotation for parasites was negative. Fecal cytology samples stained with Diff-Quik stain showed a mild elevation in both neutrophils and eosinophils. The presence of fecal eosinophils is suggestive of an eosinophilic colitis. Routine abdominal radiographs were taken and were unremarkable.

The dog was prepared for colonoscopy using multiple enemas and colonic lavage solution. Endoscopy identified an abnormal granular appearance to the mucosal surface. There was a lack of the normal-appearing submucosal blood vessels, suggesting mucosal infiltration. The mucosa was quite friable and bled easily when touched. Normal colonic mucosa should be quite resistant to endoscope trauma. Multiple colonic mucosal biopsies were obtained while withdrawing the endoscope from the colon. Histopathology confirmed an eosinophilic colitis.

Outcome

The cause of the eosinophilic colitis was undetermined. The dog was initially treated with febendazole for possible parasites. Dietary trials were then instituted for suspected food allergies. A lack of response to both anthelmintic and dietary trials required institution of prednisolone therapy. The dog clinically improved with the therapy.

Comment

Eosinophilic colitis generally responds well to therapy using either hypoallergenic diets and or corticosteroids. Gastrointestinal parasites must always be eliminated first, however.

Case 18

SIGNALMENT: 11-year-old castrated male German shepherd-mix dog

HISTORY: The dog was presented for severe tenesmus of several weeks' duration. Multiple times throughout the day, the dog would strain to defecate and would pass a small ribbonlike piece of stool that was frequently blood tinged. There was no weight loss, and the appetite was good.

P.E.: The dog was alert and active. Temperature, pulse, and respiratory rate were normal. Abdominal palpation was unremarkable except for a feces-distended colon. Digital rectal examination was normal; however, the feces present was blood tinged. The prostate was small and firm.

ENDOSCOPIC FINDINGS: An endoscopic view of the distal descending colon showed a large mass obstructing the lumen (*Figure 4.30*).

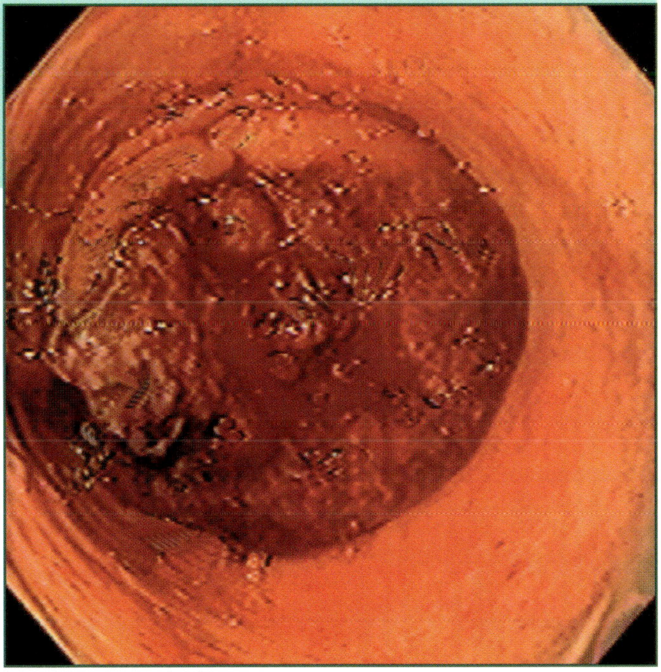

Figure 4.30 Endoscopic view of the distal descending colon showing a large hemorrhagic mass obstructing the lumen.

Initial Assessment

This dog's signs, as revealed in the history, in conjunction with physical findings of a large, distended colon, suggest a partial obstruction of the distal colon or the rectum. Differential diagnosis of colonic obstruction includes neoplasia, inflammatory polyps, strictures, and regional granulomatous lesions. Colonic neoplasia and polyps are more common in older dogs and can be associated with ulceration. Inflammatory lesions, such as fungal disease or granulomatous colitis, are possible diagnoses but are less common. Lymphocytic plasmacytic colitis, which is common in dogs, rarely, if ever, causes obstructive lesions. Colonic foreign bodies are possible but less likely than other diagnoses in this case. Neurologic abnormalities that could mimic obstructive lesions are possible but uncommon.

Presumptive Diagnosis

Colonic obstruction, possibly neoplasia, polyps, or granulomatous lesion.

Diagnostic Plan

The first diagnostic step was a good rectal examination to palpate for a cause of suspected distal colonic or rectal obstruction. No obvious lesion was identified, the prostate was small, and the fecal material was blood tinged. Fecal examination, including fecal cytology and fecal flotation, identified no abnormalities. A minimum database was obtained, including a CBC, a biochemical profile, and urinalysis. Mild microcytic anemia was identified and is consistent with an iron-deficiency anemia resulting from chronic gastrointestinal blood loss. Thoracic and abdominal radiographs were taken. Abnormalities identified included fecal distention of the transverse and descending portions of the colon and enlarged sublumbar lymph nodes. Ultrasound examination confirmed the enlarged sublumbar lymph nodes and a probable mass in the distal colon at the level of the pelvic inlet. A neoplastic colonic or rectal lesion with sublumbar lymphadenopathy from metastasis was suspected and considered likely.

The next diagnostic procedure to confirm a colonic obstructive lesion was colonoscopy. The animal was prepared for examination using multiple warm-water enemas. During colonoscopy, a large red mass (lesion) was observed obstructing the colon at the level of the pelvic inlet. The lesion was ulcerated and bled easily when touched. Multiple biopsy specimens were taken from the mass. The endoscope was passed around the lesion, but further examination of proximal colon was hampered because of residual fecal material remaining proximal to the mass. Histopathology confirmed the mass to be a colonic adenocarcinoma.

Outcome

The diagnosis of colonic adenocarcinoma with probable metastasis to the regional lymph nodes was made. A grave prognosis was given to the owners, and they elected no further diagnostics or therapy. The dog was subsequently euthanized.

Comment

Intestinal adenocarcinoma occurs most frequently in the distal colon and rectum in dogs. Associated signs are generally rectal bleeding and obstruction.

Part III

Index of Figures

Fig. 3.22....An endoscopic view of the rectum looking distally with the endoscopic tip placed in the "J position."

Fig. 3.23....An endoscopic view of the descending colon in a cat with lymphocytic plasmacytic colitis. The submucosal blood vessels cannot be seen, which is suggestive of mucosal infiltration.

Fig. 3.24....An endoscopic view of a mass located in the descending colon of a dog. Biopsy of the mass revealed colonic adenocarcinoma.

Chapter 4: Case Studies

Fig. 4.1......Esophageal stricture at the thoracic inlet in a cat.

Fig. 4.2......Using a food-barium mixture, an esophagram demonstrates luminal narrowing (arrow) at the thoracic inlet of a cat.

Fig. 4.3......Endoscopic view of an inflated balloon dilator placed in the esophageal stricture.

Fig. 4.4......Endoscopic view of the strictured area in the esophagus (*Figure 4.1*) following balloon dilation.

Fig. 4.5......Endoscopic view of the distal esophagus showing linear esophageal ulcerations, refluxed gastric contents, and an open lower esophageal sphincter.

Fig. 4.6......Endoscopic view of the distal esophagus with a bone foreign body.

Fig. 4.7......Endoscopic view of the esophagus following removal of a bone foreign body. Note the ulcerations in the esophageal wall where the bone was lodged.

Fig. 4.8......An endoscopic view of the distal esophagus and lower esophageal sphincter (LES). Dorsal to the LES is a 1.2-cm opening into a large diverticulum. Ventral to the LES is an area of ulceration from the previous bone foreign body.

Fig. 4.9......This esophagram shows retention of barium in a large esophageal diverticulum in the distal esophagus of a dog.

Fig. 4.10....Endoscopic view of the distal esophagus showing a large submucosal mass protruding into the esophageal lumen just cranial to the lower esophageal sphincter.

Fig. 4.11....An endoscopic view showing the distal esophagus of a dog with esophagitis and an open lower esophageal sphincter.

Fig. 4.12....An endoscopic view of the lower esophageal sphincter viewed from the stomach. The lower esophageal sphincter and stomach are cranially displaced through an enlarged esophageal hiatus in the diaphragm. Imprints of the esophageal hiatus can be seen on the stomach wall (arrow).

Fig. 4.13....A barium esophagram showing a dilated esophagus with the lower esophageal sphincter (arrow) and fundic portion of the stomach herniated into the thorax.

Fig. 4.14....The endoscopic view of the body of the stomach in a cat showing an irregular mucosal surface due to prominent lymphoid follicles.

Fig. 4.15....High-power oil immersion brush cytology of the gastric mucosa showing many spiral *Helicobacter* sp-like organisms (Gram's stain; ×100).

Fig. 4.16....An endoscopic view showing the gastric antrum. There is a large mucosal fold obstructing the pyloric opening.

Fig. 4.17....An endoscopic view of the body of the canine stomach showing a *Physaloptera* sp embedded in the mucosa.

Fig. 4.18....An endoscopic view showing the area of the gastric angle of the stomach. The gastric wall is rigid and thickened and has two deep mucosal ulcers.

Fig. 4.19....An endoscopic view showing the proximal duodenum of a dog. Note the prominent white villous tips of the intestinal mucosa, which are characteristic of lymphatic dilation.

Fig. 4.20....Histopathology of the duodenal mucosal biopsy showing dilated lymphatics characteristic of lymphangiectasia in the intestinal villi. (H&E stain; ×40)

Fig. 4.21....Left, The endoscopic view showing the proximal duodenum of a cat previously diagnosed to have inflammatory bowel disease. The mucosa is slightly irregular and a mucosal ulcer can be seen at approximately the 9 o'clock location in the lumen. Right, The close-up view of the duodenal ulcer in a cat with inflammatory bowel disease.

Fig. 4.22....Endoscopic view of the proximal duodenum of a dog showing hyperemic mucosa.

Fig. 4.23....Endoscopic view of the duodenum 17 cm beyond the pylorus showing narrowing of the lumen due to a white, firm, fibrouslike lesion.

Fig. 4.24....The surgically resected duodenal adenocarcinoma (arrow) was diagnosed endoscopically.

Fig. 4.25....An endoscopic view of the proximal small intestine in a cat. The mucosa has a prominent villous surface.

Fig. 4.26....Histopathology of the endoscopic biopsy showing diffuse lymphocytic lymphoma in the intestinal villi. (H&E stain; ×40)

Fig. 4.27....Endoscopic view in the proximal ascending colon showing a tissue mass projecting into the lumen. The mucosal surface of the mass appears normal.

Fig. 4.28....Endoscopic view from the colon of a dog with the endoscopic tip retroflexed into the J position viewing distally to the rectum. Two polypoid lesions are visible protruding into the rectal lumen.

Fig. 4.29....Endoscopic view of the descending colon of a dog. The mucosal surface is granular in appearance and shows a lack of normal submucosal blood vessels, suggesting mucosal inflammatory infiltrates.

Fig. 4.30....Endoscopic view of the distal descending colon showing a large hemorrhagic mass obstructing the lumen.

Glossary of Terms

-A-

antrum: the distal portion of the stomach just proximal to the pylorus and normally devoid of gastric rugae (folds).

air/water valve: a button on the endoscopic handpiece that regulates air for insufflation of the lumen and water to clean the lens on the distal tip of the endoscope.

-B-

bacterial overgrowth: a condition associated with increased bacterial concentrations in the proximal small intestine; quantitation of bacterial numbers can be made by endoscopic aspiration of duodenal fluid.

balloon dilation: a technique involving radial dilation of a luminal stricture using specialized balloons inflated by controlled pressure.

bilious vomiting syndrome: an idiopathic syndrome associated predominately with vomiting bile and believed to be related to gastric hypomotility.

biopsy forceps: endoscopic instruments used to obtain mucosal or lesion tissue. Forceps types feature either oval or serrated-edge cups.

-C-

cardia: the very proximal portion of the stomach that contains the lower esophageal sphincter.

cecal inversion: a condition in which the cecum invaginates the lumen of the colon. This condition is also referred to as a cecocolic invagination.

colonoscopy: the endoscopic technique of examining the large intestine, rectum, and cecum.

control knobs: levers on the endoscopic handpiece that control the deflection of the distal tip of the insertion tube in up/down and left/right directions.

colonic lavage solutions: iso-osmotic solutions that produce diarrhea; used to clean particulate material out of the colon prior to colonoscopy.

-D-

duodenoscopy: the endoscopic technique of examining the duodenum.

dyschezia: painful defecation.

-E-

endoscopy: the technique of examining internal body structures using specialized optical instruments. Most current endoscopes use fiberoptics for light and or image transmission.

epiphrenic: a location just cranial to the diaphragm.

esophagoscopy: the endoscopic technique of examining the esophagus.

esophageal diverticulum: a defect in the esophageal wall that results in a saclike dilatation or outpouching of mucosa through one or more layers of the wall.

-F-

fiberoptics: bundles of many small glass or plastic fibers arranged to transmit either light or an image through an optical instrument, such as an endoscope.

fecal cytology: a microscopic technique for examination of stained fecal material to determine cell types and bacteria.

fundus: the pouchlike proximal portion of the stomach adjacent to the gastric cardia.

-G-

gastric angle: the junction between the lesser curvature and pyloric antrum of the stomach. This is an important endoscopic landmark and is sometimes referred to as the gastric angulus or incisura angularis.

gastric rosette: the red color of the gastric mucosa that is sometimes seen within the lumen of the lower esophageal sphincter.

gastrinoma: an endocrine tumor, arising from the pancreatic islet cells, which secretes the hormone gastrin.

gastroesophageal junction (GEJ): the anatomic area that includes the very distal portion of the esophagus and proximal cardiac portion of stomach and contains the lower esophageal sphincter.

gastroscopy: the endoscopic technique for examining the stomach.

granlomatous enteritis: an idiopathic, chronic inflammatory condition associated with histiocytes and fibrous tissue. The lesion often extends to transmural involvement.

-H-

halogen light source: a high-intensity light source used in gastrointestinal endoscopy. This type of light often gives a slight red or yellow hue to the image.

handpiece: the working portion of the endoscope that contains the eyepiece, air/water and suction valves, control knobs, and biopsy port.

***Helicobacter* spp:** spiral, urease-producing bacteria frequently found in the stomach of dogs and cats. In some cases, *Helicobacter*-like organisms (HLO) are the cause of gastritis or gastric ulceration.

hematochezia: fresh blood in the stool.

hiatal hernia: a condition in which the cardia and a portion of the fundus slide into the thoracic cavity because of an abnormal esophageal hiatus in the diaphragm.

hypertrophic pyloric gastropathy: a condition associated with mucosal hypertrophy proximal to the pyloric canal, resulting in gastric outflow obstruction and delayed gastric emptying.

-I-

ileocolic sphincter: the anatomic muscular junction between the ileum and proximal large intestine.

incisura angularis: the gastric angle or junction between the gastric lesser curvature and pyloric antrum.

insertion tube: the long portion of the gastrointestinal endoscope that is inserted into the lumen for examination. The distal end of the insertion tube can be deflected in multiple directions by movement of the control knobs.

inflammatory bowel disease: a descriptive condition that represents a collective number of inflammatory infiltrates in both the small and large intestines.

insufflation: the process of distending the lumen of the bowel with air during an endoscopic examination.

-J-

J position: an endoscopic maneuver in which the distal tip of the endoscope is retroflexed maximally 180° or greater in the opposite direction.

-L-

leiomyoma: a benign, smooth muscle tumor frequently found in the wall of the gastrointestinal tract.

light cable: the portion of the endoscope that is attached to a light source and carries light, air, water, and suction to the endoscope. It is also referred to as the umbilical cord or light guide cable.

lumen: the interior of a tubular structure, such as the gastrointestinal tract.

lymphangiectasia: a condition of the small intestine associated with lymphatic lacteal dilation and protein-losing enteropathy.

lower esophageal sphincter (LES): the area of high pressure between the distal esophagus and stomach. Normally, the lower esophageal sphincter is closed.

-M-

megaesophagus: a condition associated with dilation of the esophagus due to abnormal esophageal motility.

-O-

odynophagia: painful swallowing.

Ollulanus tricuspis: a small gastric worm found in cats and frequently associated with chronic vomiting.

-P-

papilla, or duodenal papilla: openings where the common bile duct (major papilla) and the pancreatic duct (minor papilla) enter the duodenum in dogs. Cats have only a major duodenal papilla that contains both the pancreatic and common bile ducts entering through a common channel.

PEG: percutaneous, endoscopically placed, gastrostomy feeding tube.

***Physaloptera* sp:** a nematode parasite that is found in the stomach and proximal duodenum and is frequently associated with chronic vomiting.

polyp: a mass of mucosal tissue that projects from the luminal surface and is visible during endoscopic examination.

Peyer's patches: focal areas of lymphoid follicles located in the duodenum. Peyer's patches appear endoscopically as focal areas of depressions in the luminal wall and look much like ulcers.

pulsion diverticulum: an esophageal wall pouch or sac that develops secondary to increased esophageal intraluminal pressure.

pylorus: the muscular junction between the stomach and duodenum.

-R-

reflux esophagitis: a condition associated with esophageal mucosal ulceration secondary to reflux of gastric contents.

-S-

slide-by technique: a technique used in colonoscopy to pass the endoscope around the splenic and hepatic flexures. When using this technique, the lumen cannot be visualized.

suction valve: a button on the endoscopic handpiece that, when depressed, causes suction at the distal tip of the endoscope.

-T-

tenesmus: painful defecation.

-V-

video endoscope: an endoscope that incorporates a small video chip at the tip of the insertion tube and produces an electronic image that is then viewed on a video monitor.

-X-

xenon light source: a high-intensity light source recommended for gastrointestinal endoscopy and photo documentation. This light produces true-color images and is the recommended light source for endoscopy.

Suggested Reading

Baez JL, Hendrick MJ, Walker LM, et al. Radiographic, ultrasonographic and endoscopic findings in cats with inflammatory bowel disease of the stomach and small intestine: 33 cases (1900-1997). *J Am Vet Med Assoc.* 1999;215:349.

Burrows CF. Evaluation of a colonic lavage solution to prepare the colon of the dog for colonoscopy. *J Am Vet Med Assoc.* 1989;195:1719.

Callan MB, Washabau RJ, Saunders HM, et al. Congenital esophageal hiatal hernia in the Chinese shar-pei dog. *J Vet Intern Med.* 1993;7:210.

Chacon MB, Uson JM, Vives MA, et al. Gastroesophageal reflux in canine clinical practice. *Eur J Comp Gastroenterol.* 1999;4:25.

Church EM, Mehlhaff CJ, Patnaik AK. Colorectal adenocarcinoma in dogs: 78 cases (1973-1984). *J Am Vet Med Assoc.* 1987;191:727.

Fondacaro JV, Richter KP, Carpenter JL, et al. Feline gastrointestinal lymphoma: 67 cases (1988-1996). *Eur J Comp Gastroenterol.* 1999;4:5.

Guilford WG. Gastrointestinal endoscopy. In: Guilford WG, Center SA, Strombeck DR, et al, eds. *Small Animal Gastroenterology.* 2nd ed. Philadelphia, Pa: WB Saunders Co; 1996:114-129.

Harai BH, Johnson SE, Sherding RG. Endoscopically guided balloon dilation of benign esophageal strictures in 6 cats and 7 dogs. *J Vet Intern Med.* 1995:9:332.

Jergens AE, Moore FM, Haynes JS, Miles KG. Idiopathic inflammatory bowel disease in dogs and cats: 84 cases (1987-1990). *J Am Vet Med Assoc.* 1992;201:1603.

Jergens AE, Moore FM, March P, Miles KG. Idiopathic inflammatory bowel disease associated with gastroduodenal ulceration-erosion: a report of nine cases in the dog and cat. *J Am Anim Hosp Assoc.* 1992;28:21.

Jones BD. Endoscopy of the lower gastrointestinal tract. *Vet Clin North Am Small Anim Pract.* 1990;5:1229.

Kull PA, Hess RS, Craig LE, et al. Clinical, clinicopathologic, radiographic and ultrasonographic characteristics of intestinal lymphangiectasia in dogs: 17 cases (1996-1998). *J Am Vet Med Assoc.* 2001;219:197.

Leib MS. Chronic colitis in dogs. In: Bonagura JD, ed. *Kirk's Current Veterinary Therapy XIII.* Philadelphia, Pa: WB Saunders Co; 2000:643-647.

Leib MS, Dalton MN, King SE, Zajac AM. Endoscopic aspiration of intestinal contents in dogs and cats: 394 cases. *J Vet Intern Med.* 1999;13:191.

Leib MS, Saunders GK, Moon ML, et al. Endoscopic diagnosis of chronic hypertrophic pyloric gastropathy in dogs. *J Vet Intern Med.* 1993;7:335.

Lobetti R, Leisewitz A. Gastroesophageal reflux in two cats. *Feline Pract.* 1996;24:5.

Matthiesen DT, Walter MC. Surgical treatment of chronic hypertrophic pyloric gastropathy in 45 dogs. *J Am Anim Hosp Assoc.* 1982;22:241.

Matz ME, Leib MS, Monroe WE, et al. Evaluation of atropine, glucagon, and metoclopramide for facilitation of endoscopic intubation of the duodenum in dogs. *Am J Vet Res.* 1991;52:1948.

McCrackin MA, DeNovo RC, Bright RM, Toal RL. Endoscopic placement of a percutaneous gastroduodenostomy feeding tube in dogs. *J Am Vet Med Assoc.* 1993;203:792.

McPherron MA, Withrow SJ, Seim HB, Powers BE. Colorectal leiomyomas in seven dogs. *J Am Anim Hosp Assoc.* 1992;28:43.

Melendez LD, Twedt DC, Weyrauch EA, Willard MD. Conservative therapy using balloon dilation for intramural, inflammatory esophageal strictures in dogs and cats: a retrospective study of 23 cases (1987-1997). *Eur J Comp Gastroenterol.* 1998;3:31.

Melendez LD, Twedt DC. Suspected doxycycline induced esophagitis with esophageal stricture formation in three cats. *Feline Pract.* 2000;28:10.

Michels GM, Jones BD, Huss BT, Wagner-Mann C. Endoscopic and surgical retrieval of fishhooks from the stomach and esophagus in dogs and cats. *J Am Vet Med Assoc.* 1995;207:1194.

Miller WW, Hathcock JT, Dillon AR. Cecal inversion in eight dogs. *J Am Anim Hosp Assoc.* 1984;20:1009.

Rodriguez A, Rodriguez F, Pena L, et al. Eosinophilic gastroenteritis syndrome in a dog. *Vet Q.* 1995;17:34.

Rolfe DS, Twedt DC, Seim HB. Chronic regurgitation of vomiting caused by esophageal leiomyoma in three dogs. *J Am Anim Hosp Assoc.* 1994;30:425.

Roth L, Leib MS, Davenport DJ, Monroe WE. Comparisons between endoscopic and histologic evaluation of the gastrointestinal tract in dogs and cats: 75 cases (1984-1987). *J Am Vet Med Assoc.* 1990;196:635.

Roth L, Walton AM, Leib MS, Burrows CF. A grading system for lymphocytic plasmacytic colitis in dogs. *J Vet Diagn Invest.* 1990;4:257.

Simpson KW, Strauss-Ayali D, McDonough PL, et al. Gastric function in dogs with naturally acquired gastric *Helicobacter* spp. infection. *J Vet Intern Med.* 1999;13:507.

Stanton ME, Bright RM. Gastroduodenal ulceration in dogs. *J Vet Intern Med.* 1989;3:238.

Tams TR. *Textbook of Small Animal Endoscopy.* 2nd ed. St Louis, Mo: Mosby; 1999.

Theisen SK, LeGrange SN, Johnson SE, et al. *Physaloptera* infection in 18 dogs with intermittent vomiting. *J Am Anim Hosp Assoc.* 1998;34:74.

Twedt DC. Endoscopy case of the month: regurgitation in a puppy due to a hiatal hernia. *Vet Med.* 1993;Sept:830.

Twedt DC. Perspectives on gastrointestinal endoscopy. *Vet Clin North Am Small Anim Pract.* 1993;23:481.

Wilcock B. Endoscopic biopsy interpretation in canine or feline enterocolitis. *Semin Vet Med Surg Small Anim.* 1992;7:162.

Willard MD, Weyrauch EA. Esophagitis. In: Bonagura JD, ed. *Kirk's Current Veterinary Therapy XIII.* Philadelphia, Pa: WB Saunders Co; 2000:607-610.

Willard MD, Lovering SL, Cohen ND, Weeks BR. Quality of tissue specimens obtained endoscopically from the duodenum of dogs and cats. *J Am Vet Med Assoc.* 2001;219:474.

Williams DW. Malabsorption, small intestinal bacterial overgrowth and protein-losing enteropathy. In: Guilford WG, Center SA, Strombeck DR, et al, eds. *Small Animal Gastroenterology.* 2nd ed. Philadelphia, Pa: WB Saunders Co; 1996:367-380.

Yamasaki K, Suematsu H, Takahashi T. Comparison of gastric and duodenal lesions in dogs and cats with and without lymphocytic-plasmacytic enteritis. *J Am Vet Med Assoc.* 1996;209:95.

Zoran DL. Gastroduodenoscopy in the dog and cat. *Vet Clin North Am Small Anim Pract.* 2001;31:631.

Subject Index